Communicating Health

Communicating Health

Strategies for Health Promotion

edited by
Nova Corcoran

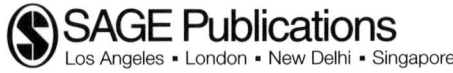

SAGE Publications
Los Angeles · London · New Delhi · Singapore

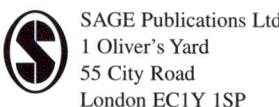 SAGE Publications Ltd
1 Oliver's Yard
55 City Road
London EC1Y 1SP

SAGE Publications Inc.
2455 Teller Road
Thousand Oaks, California 91320

SAGE Publications India Pvt Ltd
B 1/11 Mohan Cooperative Industrial Area
Mathura Road, New Delhi 110 044
India

SAGE Publications Asia-Pacific Pte Ltd
33 Pekin Street#02-01
Far East Square
Singapore 048763

British Library Cataloguing in Publication data

A catalogue record for this book is available from the British Library

ISBN 978-1-4129-2402-3
ISBN 978-1-4129-2403-0 (pbk)

Library of Congress Control Number available

Typeset by C&M Digitals (P) Ltd., Chennai, India
Printed in Great Britain by The Cromwell Press Ltd, Trowbridge, Wiltshire
Printed on paper from sustainable resources

Contents

List of figures

List of contributors

Anthony Bone works as a Principal Lecturer in Health Studies at the University of East London. He has a background in higher education, and an interest in health and social policy.

Nova Corcoran works as a Senior Lecturer in Health Promotion and Public Health at the University of East London. She has a background in health promotion work, in particular the planning, design and delivery of health campaigns and programmes.

Sue Corcoran is Assistant Director of Nursing at the Royal Cornwall Hospitals Trust. She has worked in a variety of settings in nursing and midwifery in primary and acute care, higher education and senior NHS management.

John Garlick is a Principal Lecturer in Health Service Management at the University of East London. He has worked extensively on health care policy development and on service delivery in central government and at local level in North East London.

Barbara Goodfellow works as a Senior Lecturer in Medical Sociology at the University of East London. She has a nursing background and her particular interests are inequalities in health, especially those relating to culture, gender and old age.

Calvin Moorley is a Graduate Teaching Assistant/Doctoral Student at the University of East London. His main interests are in how culture influences health and the meaning of illness. He comes from a nursing background, with a critical and primary care specialism.

Editor's acknowledgements

I would like to thank Cornwall and the Isles of Scilly Health Promotion Department who gave me my first chance to be a health promoter, my friends and colleagues at the University of East London for all their support and contributions and all the health studies students at the University of East London who gave me the idea for this book. I would like to thank Sage Publication for orientating me in the right direction, and finally I wish to thank all my friends and family, especially Ben Scott, who have had to put up with me ignoring them for months.

Nova Corcoran

Publisher's acknowledgements

Every effort has been made to trace all the copyright holders, but if any have been inadvertently overlooked the publishers will be pleased to make the necessary arrangement at the first opportunity.

The Samaritans for Figure 4.4: The Samaritans' 2002 'Change our Minds' campaign © Samaritans 2002 and Figure 5.1: The Samaritans' 2006 'txt Samaritans 4 emotional support' campaign © Samaritans 2002.

The UK Department of Trade and Transport (DfTT) for Figure 4.2: THINK! Road Safety Hedgehogs Campaign for Children.

Cancer Research for Figure 2.2: SunSmart poster reproduced by kind permission of Cancer Research ©.

Trent RDSU for Figure 8.3: Cost-effectiveness, cost-benefit and cost-utility analysis and Figure 8.6: Personal and organizational reasons for evidence-based dissemination.

J. Peterson for her suggestions to Figure 6.2: The seven key elements beneficial to establishing programmes, adapted from the original Peterson et al. (2002) work.

Sage Publications for Figure 1.6: The health belief model, Figure 1.9: Information–persuasion matrix and Figure 7.10: The steps for inculsion of evidence-based practice.

Introduction

Nova Corcoran

Health promotion is a 'dynamic, planned and measurable process' (CCP 2003) and is used to prevent morbidity and mortality and to promote a notion of holistic health and wellbeing. Communication is at the forefront of the achievement of health promotion objectives. Health practitioners have an important role in the improvement of individual, group, or community health by 'encouraging people to commence or increase health promoting behaviours and to cease or decrease health damaging behaviours' (Jones and Donovan 2004: 1).

From one-to-one contact to large-scale mass media campaigns, the promotion of health and wellbeing is underpinned by effective communication (Minardi and Riley 1997). However, communication in health promotion is not a simple linear process of providing information for immediate benefit – an assumption that has frequently been made (Lee and Garvin 2003). Assuming that communication is a linear process implies that it is a one-way information flow where a message from one source automatically translates to a behaviour change of the receiver. Health practitioners over time have come to realize that good communication in health is actually the movement towards two-way communication. Lee and Garvin (2003) refer to this as a move away from 'monologue' to 'dialogue'; in other words, moving from information transfer (a one-sided approach) to information exchange (a multi-way approach) and the concurrent reflection in health – the move from individual health education to holistic health promotion.

Daily there are new challenges to (and in) the field of health promotion and health education. Health practitioners are faced with new challenges to prevent ill health and promote preventive behaviours in response to changing patterns of mortality and morbidity worldwide. This can often be in situations where the need for health promotion outstretches budgets and resources. One premise underpinning health promotion is that all practitioners have good communication skills to enable them to promote health through the the design, planning, implementation and evaluation of programmes, campaigns or policies.

Fundamentally *Communicating Health: Strategies for Health Promotion* aims to bring together health promotion and health communication by fusing the link between theory and practice. There are thousands of health campaigns in the UK and worldwide, covering a range of topics. What is lacking is accessible information to enable clear and effective communication strategies to achieve the goals of health promotion (for example, a reduction in morbidity or a rise in those who are physically active). This textbook seeks to try and fill this 'communication gap' in the literature; its premise is that there is little use having a detailed theoretical knowledge base but few skills to implement this knowledge into practice. Likewise, there is little use having the practical skills without the theoretical rationale. If health practitioners continue to work without this fusing of theory and practice, there is a danger of practice becoming at best ineffective, at worst health damaging.

Communicating Health: Strategies for Health Promotion retains a strong academic focus, allowing practitioners to gain practical theoretical knowledge using a mixture of activities and case studies. It is aimed at the wide audience in the health promotion nexus. Health promotion is a multi-disciplinary field attracting practitioners from a range of areas. This includes the overarching fields of health promotion, health education and public health, for example, practioners in environmental health, communities, schools, hospitals, workplaces can all be engaged in health promotion work. This book is also aimed at those who are studying to become health practitioners from the range of disciplines that make up health promotion, including health studies, public health, nursing and other professions allied to medicine.

The text is presented in eight chapters. It commences with content on theoretical models and target groups and logically progresses through key topics to conclude with a chapter on evaluation. The chapters aim to take into account the range of areas that practitioners will encounter when planning, delivering and evaluating programmes, policies and campaigns. Each chapter has a number of activities. The activity discussions are found at the back of the book and are designed to give the reader examples of model answers for these activities. There is also a glossary at the end of the book, and all terms have been highlighted in the text at their first appearance. The symbol ▸▸ also appears in the margin.

Chapter 1 examines the theories and models that are used in communicating health promotion messages. This chapter provides an overview of both stage-step and cognitive theories. These theories are critiqued and applied to practical situations in a variety of different contexts. Readers are encouraged to explore the theoretical frameworks and apply these to case studies and activities.

Chapter 2 explores the social and psychological factors that are associated with target groups when planning communication campaigns. This is an area that is often overlooked in planning community strategies. This chapter seeks to highlight factors that a health practitioner should be aware of when pre-planning communication campaigns.

Chapter 3 engages with the social and cultural aspects of target groups, drawing on three hard-to-reach groups. These are different cultural groups, people living with a disability and older people. This chapter considers ways to communicate with these groups, taking into account their diversity.

Chapter 4 highlights the role of mass media in health communication, and identifies current uses of mass media. Topics include examining the role of visual and print media, utilizing the media for free and social marketing principles. This chapter seeks to enable practitioners to think critically about mass media and consider ways they can use mass media in their work more effectively.

Chapter 5 explores information technology (IT), including current use and future application to health. The role of the Internet, mobile phones and other multi-media IT in health is critiqued. Problems linked to IT in health and ways to overcome these are explored. Other issues that are covered include website design, tailoring information and Internet advocacy.

Chapter 6 examines the settings-based approach from a non-traditional perspective. Frequently, health practitioners will be working in settings to deliver health promotion work. This chapter explores the settings approach, using personal care locations (barbers, beauty salons), places of worship, universities and travel centres. These settings, which deviate from the usual settings focus, help to demonstrate the versatility of settings for health communication work.

Chapter 7 examines evidence-based practice with the premise that it is essential to the design of health promotion work. This chapter focuses on how a practitioner can use the evidence base in their work, including in the replication and location of appropriate interventions.

Chapter 8 analyses the role of evaluation in health communication. This chapter will examine the rationale for evaluation of heath promotion. It will consider strategies and methods of evaluation that can be used to illustrate effectiveness of work and the achievement of campaign goals.

On a last note, much of the research for this book has come from journals and health promotion organizations in the UK and worldwide, drawing on areas that are being constantly updated (for example, IT) where reliance on current information is essential. It is hoped that *Communicating Health: Strategies for Health Promotion* will open the debate around communication in the design of programmes, campaigns and policies to promote health, and thus move closer to achieving fundamental health promotion goals of achieving health for all.

Theories and models in communicating health messages

Nova Corcoran

Learning objectives:

- Define the term 'communication' and identify components of the communication process in a health promotion context.
- Explore communication theory in relation to health promotion practice.
- Apply theoretical models of health promotion to the health promotion and health education setting.

Communication has an essential role in any action that aims to improve health. It is difficult to imagine how a message could be delivered to promote healthy choices if we could not communicate. The communication process is a multi-dimensional transaction influenced by a variety of factors. In health promotion work the successful exchange of information between the practitioner and target audience is an area that has received mixed attention. Most commonly the emphasis on theory is clear, but the application of theory to practice is limited. This chapter introduces five theoretical models that can be applied to health promotion work. This chapter will seek to bridge the theory–practice gap using a range of examples, enabling the practitioner to link theoretical models to practice.

COMMUNICATION DEFINED

Communication is a transactional process and in a health context it is an important part of health promotion work. Communication, according to Minardi and Riley (1997) is an essential, instrumental and purposeful process. The communication transaction is one of sharing information using a set of common rules (Northouse and Northouse 1998). In *health promotion* communication is a planned process (Kiger 2004). The effectiveness of this planned process comes to fruition when the audience has achieved, acted on or responded to a message.

COMPONENTS OF COMMUNICATION

The basic representative *model* of communication is usually conceptualized as a one-way flow process consisting of a sender, message and receiver (see Figure 1.1).

   In addition to this, fourth and fifth variables can be added: complete understanding by that receiver and feedback to the communicator. These last two variables are important for health communication as they imply two-way communication, thus moving away from the traditional concept of one-way communication towards multi-way communication. It is also important to remember that communication is a cyclic process involving a series of actions, thus a modified model can be represented as circular (see Figure 1.2).

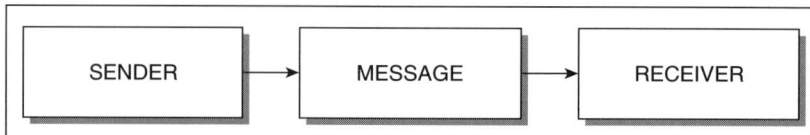

Figure 1.1   The sender, message and receiver process

FACTORS INFLUENCING COMMUNICATION

The multi-dimensional and dynamic nature of communication means that transactions contain other aspects that influence communication. Watzlawick et al. (1967) break communication down into 'content' and 'relationship'. The 'content' includes the message, the words and the information transmitted. The 'relationship' consists of the dynamics between those involved in the communication transaction – the communicator(s). This breakdown has the advantage of identifying the content and the relationship between the sender and receiver separately. In *Communicating Health: Strategies for Health Promotion* the main sender is the health practitioner and the receiver is the intended audience (who will be discussed in more detail in Chapter 2). The content aspect is currently of considerable interest in this chapter.

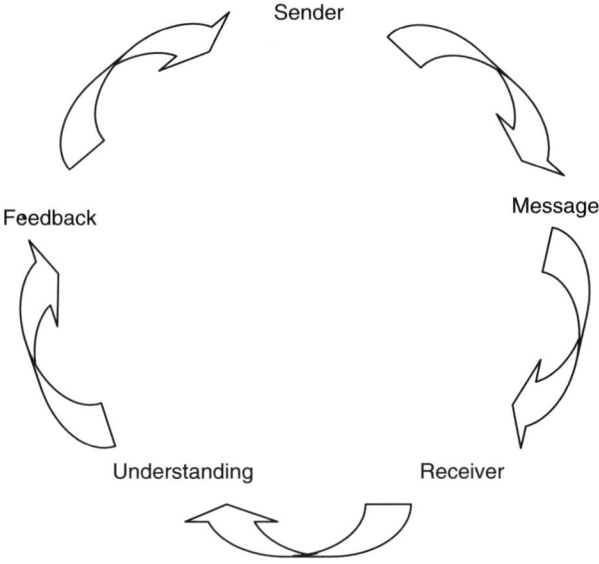

Figure 1.2   Communication as a multi-way process

The content of a message contains verbal and non-verbal communication. Verbal communication is the words, sentences and phrases used (Minardi and Reily 1997). Non-verbal communication, according to Ellis and Beattie (1986), contains the four elements of *prosodic*, paralinguistic, kinesics and standing features:

- *Prosodic elements* include intonation and rhythm. These can influence how the sender delivers the message and the receiver interprets it. For example, comprehension would alter if the sender of a message spoke quickly or slowly.
- *Paralinguistic features* include vocal but non-verbal expressions like 'mmm' or 'ahhh'. These can alter the way messages are communicated, particularly in relation to the prosodic features described above.
- *Kinesic elements* include body language, eye contact, posture or gestures. For example, different interpretations of messages would be transmitted by a sender who was trying to maintain eye contact as opposed to a sender who was looking at their feet.
- *Standing features* include factors such as appearance. Some people have pre-conceived notions of what practitioners who deliver health information should look like. This can include their dress, gender, ethnic group and other appearance-related factors.

Language and lexical content of the message is also important. Lexical content, which literally means the words, can be used positively or negatively. Using words from complex medical technology or abbreviating key terms can confuse messages and exclude the target audience, whereas using repetition has been positively found to influence communication (Pechmann and Reibling 2000).

As a health practitioner, the communication method will alter the importance of additional factors such as lexical content and body language. The communication

▶▶ process will dictate the aspects that are the most important. If you are sending every house in one area an information document about *prevention* of food-related illness and hence have minimal contact with the client group, your appearance and eye contact will be of little importance. If you are delivering a brief one-to-one intervention on stopping smoking in a health care setting your verbal communication, eye contact or appearance will be important.

COMMUNICATION IN HEALTH PROMOTION

Communication in health takes place on many levels, including individual, group, organization, community or mass-media. Communication in health can be defined in much the same way as communication has generally been defined: a transactional process. The main difference in communicating health is that the focus is not a general one but one specific to health information. Kreps (2003) summarizes the addition of 'health' to the definition of communication as a 'resource' that allows health messages (for example prevention, risk or awareness) to be used in the education and avoidance of ill health. This broad definition incorporates the fact that
▶▶ health communication can take place at many levels and embodies a *holistic* approach to health promotion.

Activity 1.1:   How are health promotion messages communicated?

There are a number of ways (or 'mediums') that can be used for communicating messages. Many of these can be used in communicating health messages.

1 Think of as many ways of communicating information as you can.
2 Which methods are most popularly used in communicating health promotion messages?

Communication methods can be divided into one of five categories: intrapersonal, interpersonal, organizational, community and public/mass communication. Figure 1.3 illustrates these five hierarchical categories and gives examples of the type of communication methods that can be included in these categories. 'Intrapersonal' incorporates internal communication. This includes what we think or listen to internally. 'Interpersonal' communication is communication on a personal level. This includes one-to-one communication or small group communication. 'Organizational' communication includes communication in an organization, both formal and informal. 'Community' communication includes mediums that are used in community settings, for example local radio and newspapers. 'Public/Mass' communication is large-scale and includes national and international communication.

Communication category	Example of communication medium
Intrapersonal	Internal communication (for example, what we think, when we listen to an inner voice)
Interpersonal	One-to-one, small groups, emails, telephone calls and other activities that allow personal listening and response
Organizational	Lectures, seminars, debates, meetings, memos, intranets, newsletters, workshops, displays
Community	Local radio, talks, seminars, debates, local newspapers, bill boards, bus wraps, health fairs
Public/Mass	Newspapers, television, digital television, national radio, Internet, CD-ROMs, mobile phones

Figure 1.3   Communication in five categories

MODELS AND THEORIES OVERVIEW

The UK government *Choosing health: making healthy choices easier* white paper (DOH 2004) identifies one fundamental and important problem with health messages: that it is not a lack of information in health, but that it is 'inconsistent, uncoordinated and out of step' (DOH 2004: 21) with the way the population live their lives. This suggests perhaps that despite efforts from health practitioners, some messages are not as effective as they could be.

The Population Reference Bureau (2005) in the US suggests that human behaviour is the central factor in most leading causes of *mortality* and *morbidity*. They advocate that behaviour change strategies should be at the forefront of any attempts to reduce mortality and morbidity. Being able to predict behaviour makes it easier to plan an intervention (Naidoo and Wills 2000). Therefore the first stage of any communication *campaign* is to analyse the behavioural aspects of the health problem (Atkin 2001).

In addition it is proposed that if we can understand factors that influence behaviour 'we will be in a better position to devise strategies and formulate methods that will achieve our *health education* goals – no matter what our philosophy or what model we choose to follow' (Tones and Tilford 1994: 83). *Theory* enables the practitioner to predict the outcomes of interventions and the relationships between internal and external variables. Underpinning communication in health promotion should be an understanding of how and why people change their behaviours and at what point of intervention it is best to target a message. This allows identification of the actions needed to change that behaviour and highlights the pathways of influence that hinder (or promote) that behaviour.

Theories do not specifically identify an intervention to follow. Instead they generate a series of ideas for a theory-led intervention to adopt. There are several theoretical models that identify influences in the behavioural change process. These are then selected according to what the practitioner wishes to achieve. The purpose of theory is to enable the successful exchange of information between the health promoter and the target audience (for example, the individual, group, population). The success of this process is often down to the influence of a number of variables. These include, for example, the relationship between the communicator and audience (as described earlier), the message itself, how the message is sent and the audiences' beliefs, values, attitudes. Theory can therefore help predict and explain behaviours, assist in the targeting of information and predict the effect that information will have. It also allows practitioners to predict why the audience may not undertake a behaviour no matter how much assistance or encouragement is available.

Theory is often used to inform the groundwork for health promotion, but is usually given less attention (if any at all) during the implementation of programmes (Kobetz et al. 2005). For example, a study by Abraham et al. (2002) examined health promotion messages in safer sex promotion leaflets. They found that the majority of the leaflets examined did not include, or refer to, messages that targeted cognitions and actions that are most strongly related to condom use. This highlights a clear gap between the evidence-based research and practice in relation to designing safer sex promotion leaflets.

The application of theory to practice is not an easy step. Health promotion in the past has made use of theory sporadically, and often inconsistently. Jones and Donovan (2004) argue that practitioners frequently ignore theory, failing to use and implement theory-based interventions. They suggest that practitioners lack the skills and knowledge needed to operationalize the generic theories and models available. This is not to say that all health practitioners are ignorant of the importance and use of theory: some practitioners may have a clear theoretical knowledge but lack the time, resources, expertise or evidence base to implement their knowledge.

If communication is based on a theoretical model, some of the pitfalls associated with poor communication can be eliminated. Tones and Tilford (1994) argue that practitioners need a framework to make a clear selection of outcome indicators and to justify choice. In addition to this, it will provide a basis for best practice. In an age of cost-effectiveness alongside the move to evidence-based practice, the inclusion of theoretical models is an almost logical one. Kobetz et al. indicate that 'construction and strategic dissemination of finely tuned, theory-based health messages' (2005: 330) alongside making theory practically relevant is one of the keys to effective communication.

Activity 1.2:   Why not use theory?

1   List all the reasons that you can think of as to why a health practitioner may not use theory in their work.

WHY USE THEORETICAL MODELS?

Models are derived from a simplified version of theory and can be used to guide the development of health promotion programmes. Theories and models are 'useful in planning, implementing and evaluating interventions' (Trifiletti et al. 2005: 299). Models in health promotion usually seek to include key elements important to behaviour and decision-making processes. In health promotion and health education, models are often borrowed from areas of social psychology or health communication and applied to health contexts.

Theories are valued in the field of health promotion because of their use in explaining influences on health alongside the ability to suggest ways where individual change could be achieved (Parker et al. 2004). Effective communication strategies should be grounded in a sound theory (Airhihenbuwa and Obregon 2000). They can be used to design and plan health promotion strategies and to generate decisions and solutions, ensuring that all variables are taken into consideration (Tones and Green 2004). As Lewin surmises, 'there is nothing more practical than a good theory' (1951: 169).

PROBLEMS ASSOCIATED WITH A THEORY-BASED APPROACH

Although the evidence for using theory is difficult to refute, the use of theory is not without its problems. Tones and Green (2004) highlight the concern that theory objectifies human experience and through this process deviates from the main health promotion ethos of *holism* and *empowerment*. This ◀◀ means that a person is seen as someone who can be measured, analysed, adjusted or directed. This process opposes the idea of the person being seen as a holistic whole, and is reductionist in nature. A broader concept of theory should perhaps be taken to alleviate the narrow, mechanistic focus that theory may have. Airhihenbuwa and Obregon (2000) suggest that theoretical frameworks should be flexible and therefore applicable to different contexts. Theory should be used as a means to guide the understanding of complex behaviour, rather than a rigid model that should be followed. In addition, Parker et al. (2004) suggest that designing interventions that attempt to focus on all aspects of a model may be both daunting and unrealistic. A suggestion is to focus on certain 'leverage points' or two or three stages in a model, for example 'subjective norms' or 'intentions'. This may also be more practical for health promotion work.

The other key criticism of the theory-based approach is that structural, political and environmental factors are excluded in many theoretical models. Behaviour and influences on behaviour are altered by the wider societal context and theory often focuses on individuals only. This approach alone will not be effective without other enabling factors present to assist the facilitation of a behaviour change. It is important to remember when designing communication campaigns that supportive environments are available to facilitate change. Wider societal influences are sometimes difficult to control, for example government priorities, thus ambitions and objectives may need to be adjusted accordingly.

Activity 1.3:   The role of wider determinants of health

As a practitioner it would be difficult to advocate change without considering the wider determinants of health, for example, location of facilities, political contexts or environmental influences. It would be difficult to advocate healthy eating in older people, for example, if there were no shops nearby selling fruit and vegetables. How would you do the following?

1   Promote cycling to work when no-one has a bicycle, and appropriate funds for bicycles or cycle paths are not available?
2   Encourage children to play in fenced park areas when there are no safe outdoor places to play or the nearest park is some distance away?

THEORIES

There are a multitude of theories that can be used in the communication of health. Five theoretical models have been selected to cover a wide range of contexts for the purposes of this textbook. This is by no means definitive coverage of the theoretical models available to the health practitioner. The models chosen have been selected for their suitability and popularity in the communication of health messages and their use in designing simple messages in leaflets to large-scale *mass media* campaigns. The models selected encompass a variety of approaches that lend themselves to different communication projects in the health field.

In this chapter we will consider two types of theoretical models: cognitive theories and stage-step theories:

- *Cognitive theories* provide 'continuum accounts of behaviour' (Rutter and Quine 2002: 15), proposing that a certain set of perceptions or *beliefs* will predict a behaviour. In the cognitive theories section the *Theory of Planned Behaviour* (Ajzen 1980) and *Health Belief Model* (Becker 1974) will be examined, and applied to the health communication context.
- *Stage Step theories* assume that the individual is not on a continuum (as they are in cognitive theories) but at a 'step' or 'stage'. Each step on the model is a move forward towards achieving the behaviour. Stage-step theories postulate that the individual goes through a process of change via a series of stages. Their format can be represented as cyclic or a literal series of steps. In this section the *'transtheoretical model' or 'stages of change model'* (Prochaska and Diclemente 1983), the 'process of behavioural change' (Population Communication Services/Centre for Communication Programmes 2003) and the *'communication–persuasion* matrix' (McGuire 1976, 2001) will be explored.

THE THEORY OF PLANNED BEHAVIOUR (TPB)

This theory is the modified version of the *theory of reasoned action* (TRA) (Ajzen ◀◀
and Fishbein 1980), where the additional variable of 'perceived behavioural control' has been added. The TRA originally proposed that any intervention attempting
to change behaviour should focus on beliefs, as these influence *attitudes* and expec- ◀◀
tations and in turn influence intentions and behaviours. It was then proposed that
behaviours are *not* under 'volitional control' and the model was re-visited and
expanded to include 'perceived behaviour control' (Rutter and Quine 2002). The
TRA was revised to the *theory of planned behaviour* (TPB) (Ajzen 1991). The TPB ◀◀
follows the same hypothesis as the TRA with the addition of 'behavioural control'
as a determinant of behavioural intention and behavioural change (see Figure 1.4).

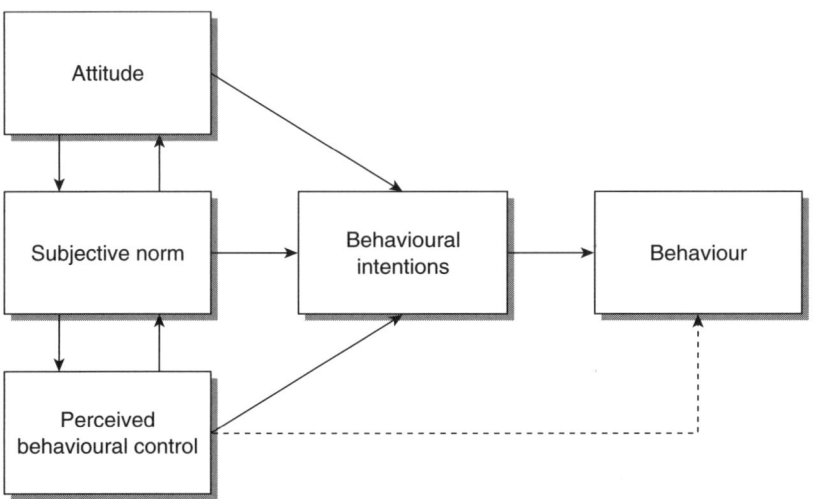

Figure 1.4   The theory of planned behaviour, adapted from Ajzen (1991)

The TPB states that the closest determinant of behaviour is the intention to perform (or not perform) that behaviour (Jackson et al. 2005; Lavin and Groarke
2005). The TPB's main determinant of behaviour is based on the person's intention to perform that behaviour, and intention is determined by three factors:

1   *Attitude to the behaviour:* the balancing of the pros/cons of performing the behaviour or the
    risks/rewards they associate with that choice.
2   *Subjective norm:* social pressure from significant others, for example peers, media or family.
3   *Perceived behavioural control:* the perception that person has about their ability to perform the
    behaviour.

This model can be represented more simplistically (see Figure 1.5). The simplistic version of the model proposes that the more positive the attitude, supportive the

subjective norm and higher the perceived behavioural control *and* the stronger the intention, the more likely it is that a person will perform that behaviour (Lavin and Groarke 2005).

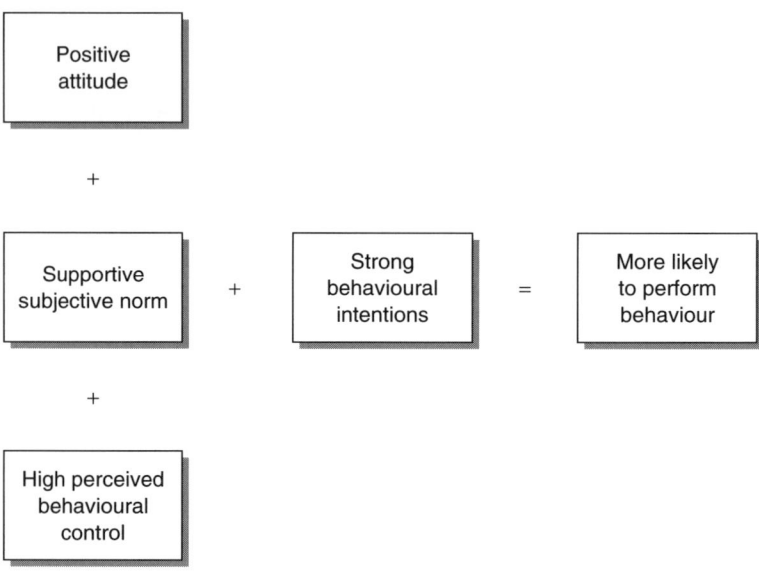

Figure 1.5   A simplistic view of the theory of planned behaviour hypothesis

---

Activity 1.4:   The theory of planned behaviour in action

Daniel has been going to the gym for a few weeks as he wants to build up his muscles to make him look good. He has noticed no improvement so far in his muscles and the gym is costing him money. Daniel gets talking to one of the staff at the gym and explains how he feels and asks for some advice. The member of staff suggests he tries taking a supplement like steroids to help him build up his muscles. The staff member says he uses steroids and he feels great, and gained muscles in 'no time'.

1   Using the theory of planned behaviour, do you think he will take the steroids?

The TPB has been widely applied in the context of understanding and predicting behaviour (Bledsoe 2005). Recently it has been used for a number of different health behaviours, including promoting walking among sedentary adults (Reger et al. 2002), smoking cessation (Bledsoe 2005), a predictor of exercise take-up (Norman et al. 2000; Kelley and Abraham 2004), exercise motivation (Papauessis et al. 2005), dental floss behaviour (Lavin and Groarke 2005) and blood donation behaviours (Giles et al. 2004).

HEALTH BELIEF MODEL

Becker (1974) developed the *health belief model* (HBM) from the work of ◀◀
Rosenstock (1966). This model can be used as a pattern to evaluate or influence
individual behavioural change. Figure 1.6 illustrates the health belief model.

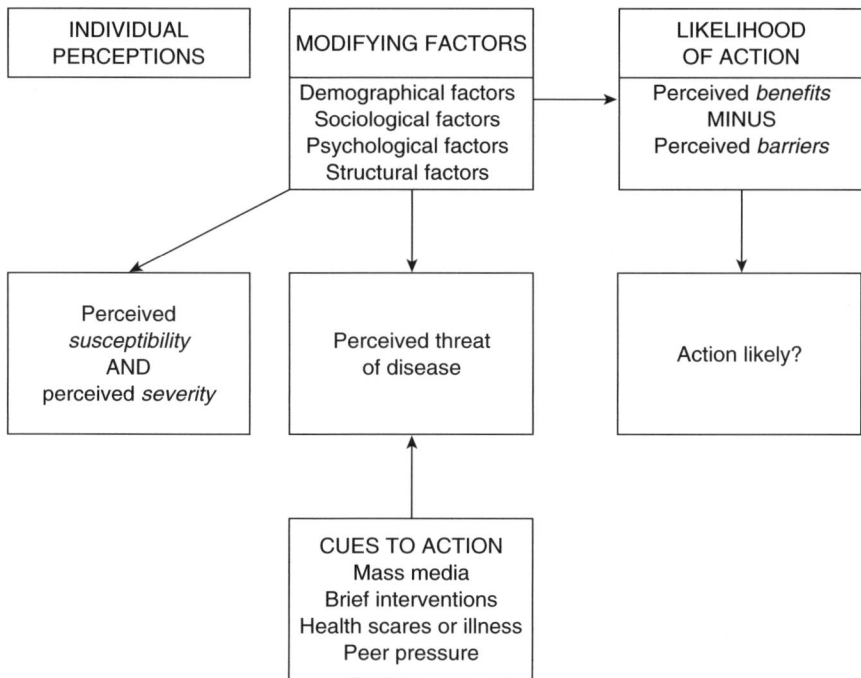

Figure 1.6 The health belief model, adapted from Rosenstock et al. (1988)

The model proposes that a person's behaviour can be predicted based on how
vulnerable the individual considers themselves to be. 'Vulnerability' is expressed
in the HBM through risk (perceived susceptibility) and the seriousness of consequences (severity). These two vulnerability variables need to be considered before
a decision can take place. This means a person has to weigh up the costs/benefits
(Naidoo and Wills 2000) or pros/cons of performing a behaviour. For example, this
could include how 'susceptible' they feel they are to contracting an illness, for
example mumps, and how 'severe' the consequences of having mumps is, or how
'susceptible' they are to an injury, for example falling off a bicycle without
protective clothing, and how 'severe' the consequence will be. A person's decision
to perform the health-promoting (or damaging) behaviour will be based on the outcome of this 'weighing up' process. Self-efficacy is also added to the HBM to
enable prediction of behaviour. Self-efficacy is a person's perceived confidence of
their ability to perform that behaviour.

The HBM includes four factors that need to take place for a behaviour change
to occur:

1 *The person needs to have an 'incentive' to change their behaviour*
   For example: An 'incentive' for a person to stop smoking could be the desire not to smoke around a new baby.
2 *The person must feel there is a 'risk' of continuing the current behaviour*
   For example: By not taking preventive measures, such as compliance with anti-malarial drugs in a high malaria risk area, a person would feel that they would be putting themselves at 'risk' of contracting malaria.
3 *The person must believe change will have 'benefits', and these need to outweigh the 'barriers'*
   For example: A person may believe that the benefits of using a bicycle helmet means they are less likely to have a serious head injury if they fall off their bicycle. They also identify the barriers to wearing one; they are cumbersome to carry throughout the day. The 'benefits' must outweigh the 'barriers' in order for a change to be made.
4 *The person must have the 'confidence' (self-efficacy) to make the change to their behaviour*
   For example: A person must believe they have the ability to cut down their fatty food intake to help them lose weight and are 'confident' about their abilities to do this.

The HBM additionally suggests that there is a 'cue to action' to prompt the behaviour change process. This could be a conversation with a friend or a television programme. Alternatively, it could be an external prompt, such as moving employment. The prompt, however, has to be appropriate to that person or, as Naidoo and Wills suggest, this cue needs to be 'salient or relevant' (2000: 225).

The HBM also considers 'modifying factors' important to behaviour change. These include demographic variables, socio-psychological variables and structural variables that influence how a person perceives the disease severity, threats and susceptibility. Factors such as age, gender, peer pressure or prior contact with the disease also impact on the decision-making process.

Case Study 1.1   The health belief model in action

Theo never wears a seatbelt. He has never crashed his car and thinks he is a good driver. He thinks seatbelts restrict his movement when driving, and none of his friends wear seatbelts either.

Outcome: Using the HBM, the benefits Theo sees of wearing a seatbelt are minimal, and the barriers to wearing one are numerous (ruins his image, restricts movement etc). It is likely that his decision will be that he does not wear a seatbelt as the costs (ruined image, restricted movement) outweigh the benefits (safety, injury prevention).

Activity 1.5:   The health belief model in action

Suki is a 10-a-day 'social' smoker. She has been sent an email about 'No Smoking Day' in March from one of her friends. She has often seen advertisements about stopping smoking, but does not think they apply to her as she is a 'social' smoker, and only smokes in the evenings when she goes out with her friends and has a drink after work. Her father has lung cancer from smoking, and is currently in hospital.

(Continued)

1   Using the health belief model, what is the likelihood that she will stop smoking
    on 'No Smoking Day' in March?
2   What health promotion advice could you give Suki?

This model, and elements from it – particularly 'perceived barriers' and 'perceived susceptibility' – has been used to predict preventive health behaviours (Naidoo and Wills 2000) and sick role behaviours (Janz and Becker 1984). Recently these have included the practice of adolescent health behaviours to prevent SARS (severe acute respiratory syndrome) (Wong and Tang 2005), sexual behaviours and risk-taking (Lin et al. 2005), choices to use public transport (Mulberry Research and Consulting Group 2004), risk of BSE (bovine spongiform encephalopathy) and dietary behaviours (Weitkunat et al. 2003), and vaccination behaviour (De Wit et al. 2005).

CRITICISMS OF COGNITIVE THEORIES

There are a number of criticisms of TPB and the HBM alongside other social cognitive models. Social cognitive models (the HBM in particular) emphasize a rational approach to behaviour and may exclude influential aspects such as friends, family or social norms. The TPB places emphasis on attitudes as a predictor of behavioural intention, but behaviour cannot necessarily be predicted by attitudes (Naidoo and Wills 2000). Careful consideration of which attitudes are more likely to lead to a behaviour intention needs additional thought. The exclusion of the wider determinants of health from social cognitive models is a frequently cited criticism. Without identification of these wider determinants, some aspects of social cognitive models may not actually determine behaviour.

Another criticism of these models is that they may be more suitable for small or high-risk populations, rather than large-scale high-risk populations (Elder 2001). The role of behavioural intentions may also be less important in non-Western cultures, as these theories assume a degree of autonomy alongside the Western biomedical model (King et al. 1995). In addition, the role of cultural contexts is missing and in non-Western populations these theories may be less culturally sensitive (Lin et al. 2005), especially if they promote individualism and remove emphasis on family or group behaviours (Airhihenbuwa and Obregon 2000). Careful examination of these aspects needs consideration before a model is chosen for use.

TRANSTHEORETICAL MODEL (TTM) (OR STAGES OF CHANGE MODEL)

The *transtheoretical model* (TTM), more frequently referred to as the 'stages of change' model, is a cyclic model developed by Prochaska and Diclemente (1983).

The model suggests that people change their behaviour at certain stages in life, rather than making one major change. During these incremental stages, they consider whether or not to make changes to their behaviour (see Figure 1.7).

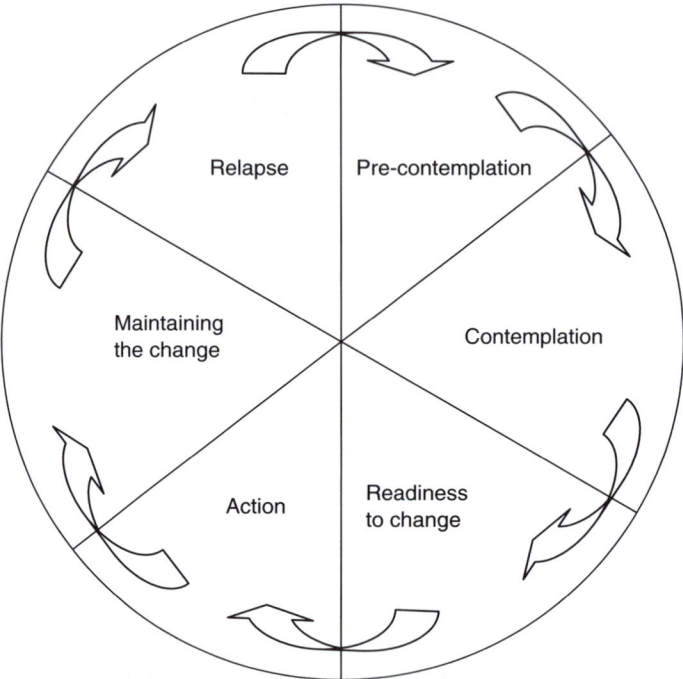

Figure 1.7   The transtheoretical model, adapted from Prochaska and Diclemente (1983)

This cyclic model is based on the premise that people are at different levels of readiness to change and during the change process they move through a series of stages. People move from *precontemplation* (not ready to change) to *contemplation* (thinking of change), to *preparation* (getting ready to change), to *action* (performing the change), to *maintenance* (continuing the change), to *relapse* (abandoning changes and reverting to former behaviours). A person may start at any of these stages and may move between stages.

Case Study 1.2   Physical activity and the transtheoretical model (TTM)

Precontemplation: A person who is sedentary and does not perceive any risks in being sedentary would be in the precontemplation phase of the TTM as they are not ready to change their behaviour yet. They cannot see any harm or risks in remaining sedentary.

Contemplation: A person who is sedentary, but is aware of the risks of being sedentary and is perhaps considering the benefits or cons of exercise would be in the contemplation stage.

Preparation: Someone who is sedentary but has gone to the local gym to sign up for aerobics classes or is planning a walking route to work, would be in the preparation stage as they are getting ready to change.

Action: A person who has started exercising and has done so for a number of weeks would be in the action phase.

Maintenance: Once the person has been performing that behaviour (usually for six months or more), they are in the maintenance stage.

Relapse: At any of these stages, a person could 'fall off' this cycle. Perhaps despite planning they started to exercise for a few weeks before stopping. At this stage the person is seen to 'relapse' and then will move backwards to another stage of the cycle.

The TTM uses are extensive and the model has frequently been used in targeting intervention programmes and *tailoring information* to appropriate stages of change. Kidd et al. (2003) indicate that the TTM could provide precision when examining effectiveness and long-term efficacy in an intervention. It has also been said that it is a model that is 'simple, powerful, discerning and practical' (Brug et al. 2005). One of the most appealing aspects of the TTM to practitioners is its simplicity. Although originally designed for smoking interventions, recently the TTM has been used in areas that include promoting fruit and vegetable consumption (Ruud et al. 2005), injury prevention (Kidd et al. 2003) and physical activity (Marshall and Biddle 2001).

Activity 1.6:   The transtheoretical model (TTM) in action

Where would you place these people on the transtheoretical model? Use Figure 1.7 to help you.

1   I now go to the dentists every 6 months for a check-up after that abscess in my tooth – it was so painful.'
2   'I have been eating healthier for the last month.'
3   'I have cycled to work for just over a year now, it's so much quicker than sitting in traffic.'
4   'Cigarettes can't kill you! My uncle lived until he was 102 and he smoked all his life.'
5   'I have joined the local gym and am going to my first class on Monday, and I have arranged for my children to be looked after by a neighbour.'
6   'I enjoy getting drunk with my friends, but my hangovers are getting worse and I would really like to have time to do more at the weekend.'

PROCESS OF BEHAVIOUR CHANGE (PBC)

▶▶   An alternative model to the TTM is the *perceived behavioural control* (PBC) model. Described by the Population Communication Services/Center for Communication Programs (2003) in the US, this model recognizes communication as a process where people can move between the stages of the PBC framework. Different messages are sought depending on where the person is on the PBC framework. The main difference between the PBC and the TTM is that the model is not seen as circular, but as a series of 'steps' where a person moves upwards towards the final goal.

In the PBC people move through the following steps:

- *Preknowledge*: when a person is unaware of any risks or problems associated with their behaviour.
- *Knowledgeable*: when a person is aware of the problem and of the risks attached to their behaviour.
- *Approving*: when a person is in favour of changing their behaviour.
- *Intending*: when a person is intending to take action to change their behaviour.
- *Practicing*: when the intended behaviour is being practiced.
- *Advocating*: when the new behaviour is being implemented and when a person then advocates that behaviour to another.

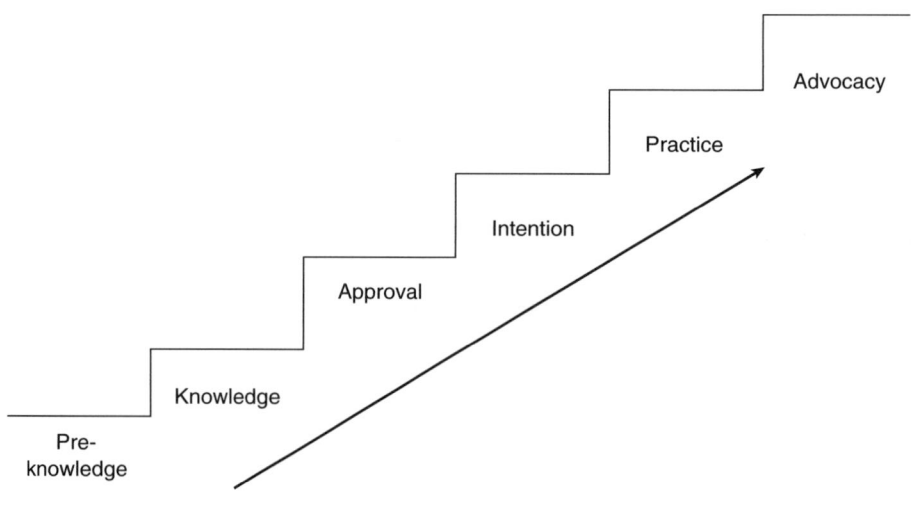

Figure 1.8   The perceived behavioural control (PBC) model, based on Population Communication Services/Center for Communication Programs

Case Study 1.3   Eating more calcium-rich foods and the perceived behavioural control (PBC) model

Preknowledge: This step is when a person is not aware they may need to eat more calcium-rich foods.

Knowledgeable: When a person has the knowledge that calcium-rich food may reduce deficiency diseases such as osteoporosis.

Approving: This step is when the person is in favour of eating more calcium-rich foods.

Intending: This step is when that person wants to change their behaviours (i.e. their diet) and intends to eat more calcium-rich foods.

Practicing: This step is when a person starts to eat more calcium-rich foods.

Advocating: The person has been practicing eating calcium-rich foods over a period of time and is advocating the behaviour (calcium-rich foods) to others.

Activity 1.7:   The perceived behavioural control (PBC) model in action

You are working in a local community and you want to raise awareness about new recycling bins that are now available for community use. You are trying to encourage those that use the recycling bins already to advocate using them to others.

1   What would people need to do at each step on the PBC model to achieve this?

CRITICISMS OF STAGE-STEP THEORIES

Stage-step models have been criticised for a number of reasons. First, people have competing priorities and therefore the behaviour (for example, stopping smoking) may not be seen as important to that person at that time (Naidoo and Wills 2000). Practitioners and the targeted individual's idea of which stage the person is in may conflict or be inaccurate (Brug et al. 2005). Some people may place themselves at wrong stages on the model, or their actions are interpreted as being in a different phase than they actually are. This may lead to limited success. West (2005) argues that some of the stages are 'soft' options, for example moving from pre-contemplation to contemplation, is not a strong move to change behaviour as there is no measurable behaviour change. West (2005) also argues that the TTM assumes that the individual has made a rational plan (for example, to quit smoking) that does not take into account entrenched habits or irrationality. Aspects included in social cognitive models, for example ▶▶ *self-efficacy*, attitudes or subjective norms, are not included in the TTM.

Brug et al. (2005) debate a variety of aspects of the TTM. They consider that it is difficult to apply to complex behaviour, especially if environmental variables are also needed to change (for example, behaviours that need money or transportation). They also argue that the TTM is more likely to change short-term behaviours than long-term. Rutter and Quine (2002) highlight a number of current debates about stage-step models, including the premise that barriers are the same for each individual at each stage. Individuals put different emphasis on different barriers (something that cognitive models recognize) and the TTM makes the assumption that these barriers will all be similar.

THE COMMUNICATION–PERSUASION MODEL AND THE INFORMATION–PERSUASION MATRIX

The communication–persuasion model (McGuire 1976, 2001) is different from other theoretical models in the health field, and its uses are predominately found in the field of advertising. The communication–persuasion model has guided ▶▶ *public health* communication particularly in using mass media (Elder 2001), which makes it different from other health promotion models that traditionally focus on small-scale, at-risk populations. This model has been used in a variety of ways. These include the examination of consumer behaviour in response to messages; for example, Kaphingst et al. (2004) use McGuire's communication–persuasion matrix to help analyse direct-to-consumer television prescription drug adverts.

McGuire is responsible for developing both an information–persuasion model (IPM) and the communication–persuasion model. The IPM can be used in conjunction with an information–persuasion matrix (McGuire 2001). According to McGuire (1976), the IPM proposes three factors that can influence a person's choice.

- *External factors,* for example price or location.
- *Internal directive factors,* for example individual attitudes or beliefs.
- *Internal dynamic factors,* for example demographic characteristics such as age or ethnicity.

The main concern of the IPM is 'internal' factors. These factors are seen to influence or change the message as it moves through the communication–persuasion model, and its progressive input–output steps.

The communication–persuasion model can be characterized as an input–output matrix that can be manipulated and measured to achieve a change. The communication 'input' factors contain five separate stages of communication: source, message, channel, receiver and destination. These input variables provide options for health practitioners to select and manipulate. These 'input' variables are the main step in achieving the 'output' variables. Figure 1.9 illustrates how McGuire has split these five 'Input' variables into sub-divisions, for example, attractiveness or non-verbal aspects.

Input Communication Factors

	INPUT	Factors in this 'input' section include:
1	Source	Demographics, credibility, attractiveness etc.
2	Message	Appeal, organization, style etc.
3	Channel	Type of media used, i.e. television
4	Receiver	Demographics, social/psychological factors
5	Destination	Immediacy/delay, prevention/cessation

Output Persuasion Techniques

	OUTPUT	Description of what happens at each step:
1	Tuning in	Exposure to the message
2	Attending	Paying attention to the message
3	Liking	Liking and being interested in the message
4	Comprehending	Understanding the message
5	Generating	Related cognitions
6	Acquiring	Gaining the appropriate skills to act on the message
7	Agreeing	Agreeing the message is correct
8	Storing	Saving the message to memory
9	Retrieval	Retrieval of the message from memory when needed
10	Decision	Acting on the message
11	Acting	Performing the action
12	Post-action	Integration of the action into behaviour
13	Converting	Advising others to behave likewise

Figure 1.9 Information–persuasion matrix, adapted from McGuire (2001)

The 13 output variables (or stages) are a sequence of events that, according to McGuire (2001), must take place in an order (1 to 13) to enable the message to have an effect and a change to happen. It is assumed that a person cannot, for example, complete step 6 (acquiring relevant skills) without first completing step 2 (attending to the communication). In some ways this is similar to the PBC model of 'steps' where the message can only be acted upon when the person has moved up the steps. McGuire is proposing that all of these stages must be completed to reach the final stages of 11 (acting on the message) to 12 (post-action cognitive integration of the behaviour) to finally 13 (proselytizing, or advocating, others to behave likewise).

Case Study 1.4   Communication–persuasion model in practice: 5 a day

1   **Tuning in**: Exposure to the five-a-day message.
2   **Attending**: Paying attention to the five-a-day message.
3   **Liking**: Liking and being interested in the message.
4   **Comprehending**: Understanding the message concept (i.e. need to eat five different types of fruit and vegetables every day).
5   **Generating**: Related cognitions (thinking what would need to be done to eat five a day.
6   **Acquiring**: Gaining skills to act on the message, for example cooking, shopping, changes to diet.
7   **Agreeing**: Agreeing to eat five a day.
8   **Storing**: Storing the five a day.
9   **Retrieval**: Being able to retrieve five a day at appropriate times (i.e. in the supermarket, when cooking).
10   **Decision**: Deciding to eat five fruit and vegetables every day.
11   **Acting**: Eating five fruit and vegetables a day.
12   **Post-action**: Continuing to eat five a day.
13   **Converting**: Encouraging or advising others to eat five a day.

Activity 1.8:   The information–persuasion matrix in action

Using Figure 1.9 to help you, what would a person need to do at each of the 1–13 stages to successfully perform the following behaviour:

1   Respond to a message that says, 'Use a condom to prevent sexually transmitted infections' (aimed at 16–18-year-olds).

The advantage of this model is that it has clear planning stages that can be followed in order to obtain an outcome. For example, Bull et al. (2001) used the communication–persuasion matrix and found that there were a number of features of printed health education materials that can lead to behaviour change in overweight adults. These include attractiveness, encouragement, levels of information and application to ones' self. These were all associated with the early steps in the communication–persuasion matrix. This suggests that these might be areas to focus on when designing health promotion materials to enable progression through the stages of the matrix. Alcalay and Bell (2000) propose that one advantage of this

module is that *evaluation* has to be included in the communication strategy as ◀◀
it is built into the model. The model can also help practitioners to identify and
consider channels and strategies that can influence the campaign outcomes. Given
the emphasis on each stage, each message stage can be examined for impact,
appropriateness and effectiveness.

CRITICISMS OF THE COMMUNICATION–PERSUASION MODEL

This model has been criticised for a number of reasons. These include having an
overly restrictive number of steps in order for a behaviour change to take place
(Scholten 1996) – the TTM and the PBC have around half this number. McGuire
(2001) himself considers that the matrix may restrict concentration on a single
variable at a time, as they all interact with one another. McGuire also considers
that the matrix assumes rational behaviour and the process of response to a message may not be a linear process. The analogy to an information processor (or
computer) is evident in the title of the model itself. As with the criticisms highlighted in the cognitive models, people do not necessarily act in a rational or logical manner, and do not process information in a rational way. Finally, Huhman
et al. (2004) suggest that as the audience processes a message, a percentage of
this audience are lost at each step. Therefore, for this model to be effective, high
exposure – and high awareness levels – are essential. The model lends itself
therefore to more high-profile, high-level communication than smaller communication efforts.

PRACTICAL IMPLICATIONS: WHICH THEORETICAL MODEL?

There are many models and theories in use in the respective disciplines of communication and health promotion. Some of these are of more use to the health
practitioner than to others. It is not simply the case that 'one model fits all'.
Communication in the health setting uses different methods, with different
messages for different audiences. All the models described (alongside some not
described – see the additional reading section at the end of this chapter) have the
potential to be utilized effectively in the communication of health promotion and
health education messages.

There are no set guidelines for practitioners to help them select which model to
use. Tones and Green (2004) list a series of questions that the practitioner could
consider before selecting models;

- Does it include all relevant variables?
- Does it make logical sense to use this model in this particular situation?
- Has it been used elsewhere for similar purposes?
- Are their any studies to illustrate its use in the chosen area?

Alongside these questions, selection of theoretical models can include personal choice, target group, funding, time, influences of stakeholders, size of project and behaviours that are being targeted. Figure 1.10 illustrates each theoretical model with the common client/person contact that it has been used for. The table also shows settings where this model has been applied and the appropriate topic interventions. This is by no means a comprehensive list of every setting or topic these models have been used for, and practitioners should investigate their own topic fully before selecting a model(s) of choice to use in their communication project.

MODEL	Client/person contact	Example settings	Examples of topic interventions
Theory of planned behaviour (TPB)	Face-to-face Groups Mass media	*Group settings* Church, schools, universities, workplaces *Wider settings* Communities, towns	• Physical activity • Accident/injury prevention • Tobacco uptake • Oral health • Alcohol/drug misuse
Health belief model (HBM)	Face-to-face Groups	*Group settings* Church, schools, universities, work places	Preventive behaviour: • Physical activity • Sexual health • Vaccinations • Dietary changes
Transtheoretical model (TTM) or perceived behavioural control (PBC)	Face-to-face Groups Self-help (i.e. via Internet)	*Medical settings* General practice, dentists, pharmacies *Group settings* Schools, universities, workplaces *Service settings* Stop smoking Groups, Screening	• Tobacco • Physical Activity • Alchol/drug misuse • Accident/injury prevention • Cancer screening • Nutrition/diet
Communication–persuasion matrix	Little or no person contact (i.e. mass media)	*Wider settings* Communities, neighbourhoods, towns, cities	Wider public health issues: • CHD • Cancer • Tobacco • Infectious disease • Prescription drugs

Figure 1.10 Examples of theoritical models that can be used in practice by group, setting and intervention

PRACTICAL IMPLICATIONS: GETTING STARTED

Often models assume some pre-contact with the client/person before an intervention can take place. For example, if you can identify the barriers that the client groups experience or the attitudes that are shared in relation to behaviours, it is easier to identify the topics to address. Communicating with your chosen target group before your intervention commences enables you to foster a more *bottom-up approach* to ◀◀ health communication, facilitating a transactional information exchange process.

However, if you cannot access the target group beforehand, this makes things more complex. How do you know that your intervention will be successful if you cannot ask any questions beforehand? Also, the planned intervention will be taking a *top-down* ◀◀ *approach*, communication will be one-sided and may exclude the very group you are trying to reach. The principles of evidence-based practice (see Chapter 7), alongside researching other campaigns in your chosen area, will be of help here.

PRACTICAL IMPLICATIONS: INDIVIDUAL CHANGE vs STRUCTURAL CHANGE

Cohen et al. (2000) argue that there are two basic targets of health interventions and all interventions can be divided into these two main targets:

- *Target one* is those interventions that seek to change individuals and in the control of individual(s).
- *Target two* is those that seek to change structures and are therefore outside of the control of the individual(s).

Interventions that use an individual approach usually want to influence or change attitudes, beliefs, knowledge or skills. Those at a structural level seek to change variables out of the individual control, for example, by adapting environments or increasing accessibility of services. Interventions can also be a combination of the two.

Case Study 1.5   Individual change and structural change

A peer education campaign in a university that aims through role play to change first year student's condom negotiation skills would be classed as having an individual change target (the change is in the control of the individual).

Structural change: A campaign that aims to increase the amount of condom machines available throughout the university would be classed as having a structural change target (the change is in the control of the authorities fitting the machines).

A combination: Individual and structural change: a campaign that aims to use peer education through role play to change students' condom negotiation skills alongside increasing the amount of condom machines available throughout the university and in first-year halls of residence.

Activity 1.9:   Individual, structural or both?

Examine the following communication projects and identify if you think they are: *Individual, Structural* or *both*.

1   A teacher-led project in a secondary school that aimed to introduce female pupils to three new types of physical activities (dance, tai-chi and yoga) to encourage positive attitudes to physical activity.
2   A video designed by a major airline to encourage chair exercise to decrease the risks of DVT on aeroplane flights screened to all passengers on flight take-off.
3   A programme run by a transport service to introduce newly designed bus services in a capital city and extend existing bus routes.

THE THEORY OF PLANNED BEHAVIOUR IN PRACTICE

Application of the TPB is particularly useful when there is access to a group first, allowing the mapping of major beliefs that may help or hinder performance of behaviours. One of the other advantages of this model is the inclusion of the 'subjective norm' allowing focus on peer or family influences. Recent campaigns have focussed on behavioural beliefs, normative beliefs and perceived behavioural control. Stead et al. (2005) give an overview of the 'Fools speed' driving campaign in Scotland in 1999–2001. The intervention aimed to target behavioural beliefs, normative beliefs and perceived behavioural control. Behavioural control messages focused on the consequences of speeding, for example, causing an accident. Normative beliefs focused on how others perceived speeding, and perceived behavioural control was used to remind drivers that they could control their own speed. Case Study 1.6 illustrates the theory of planned behaviour in action in a different context (physical activity).

Case Study 1.6   Theory of planned behaviour in action

The campaign 'Wheeling walks' in West Virgina (Reger et al. 2002) utilized a variety of strategies to promote walking among sedentary adults. In order to identify physical activity and walking habits, they used a telephone survey questionnaire alongside behavioural observation measurements to literally count the number of walkers. They used the TPB (and the TTM) to encourage behaviour change. In their use of the TPB they identified one barrier as an 'I don't have time' belief. They selected this as the basis for their advertisements and focussed on suggestions for starting low, for example 10 minutes a day compared to the 30 minutes a day of a television programme. The concluding statement was 'Isn't it time you started walking', hence challenging the 'I don't have time' belief.

THE HEALTH BELIEF MODEL IN PRACTICE

The health belief model can be applied to a variety of health behaviours. Interventions using this model usually aim to influence the 'perceived threat of disease' variable and hence change the susceptibility/severity balance. The main way of doing this tends to be directing information that has an emotional appeal or contains a strong fear or emotional response. Topics such as drink-driving, accidents, domestic violence, substance misuse (particularly illegal drugs) and road safety are good examples of this and often lend themselves to creating an emotional response to the topic (see Chapter 4 for more on this).

As the health belief model suggests that barriers may be more important than benefits (Lajunen and Räsänen 2004; Janz and Becker 1984), barriers may also provide a focus for targeting communication. For example, studies indicate that concern about pain in *screening* for preventive behaviours (Bryd et al. 2004; ◀◀ Weinberg et al. 2004, in colon and cervical screening) can be a significant barrier to overcome. If a practitioner can identify barriers to performing behaviours, an intervention can focus on these to promote a behaviour change.

Other aspects of the HBM have also been found to be associated with behaviours. Moser et al. (2005) found perceived benefits to be a predictor of fruit and vegetable consumption. Lin et al. (2005) suggests that self-efficacy is a strong predictor of sexual behaviour, whereas Weltkunat et al. (2003) found 'perceived threat' important to an aspect of dietary behaviour. De Wit (2005) promotes the use of perceived susceptibility and severity as being important components of interventions, thus illustrating that 'part's of the TPB could be used in practice'. See Case Study 1.7 for an example of perceived severity/susceptibility in action.

Case Study 1.7   The health belief model (HBM) in practice – asthma

A Community Action Against Asthma (CAAA) example (Parker et al. 2004).

As part of the CAAA, the HBM was used to target information to children with asthma and their care-givers, given by a community environmental specialist (CES). Education messages were aimed at increasing *perceived susceptibility* and increasing the care-givers *perceived severity* by identifying with the care-givers different types of environmental allergens or irritants and how they can affect children's asthma. To increase care-givers' *perceived benefits,* the CES practitioner explained links between reducing environmental allergens or irritants and ways to do this (cleaning etc.) and the benefit to the child. In response to *perceived barriers,* provision of vacuum cleaners, cleaning supplies, mattress covers etc. were made available alongside referral to appropriate agencies to help with issues such as childcare.

APPLICATION OF THE TRANSTHEORETICAL MODEL (TTM) TO PRACTICE

Application of the TTM (or the PBC) is particularly useful when there is access to the client group first allowing the mapping of individuals to stages, preferably through face-to-face involvement. For example, the TTM provides an opportunity for stage-tailored information, such as tailoring newsletters (Ruud et al. 2005) or brief advice. First, questions will need to be asked of the client. These should include questions about past behaviour, current behaviour and future intentions, including current knowledge and practice. The questions can be brief and allow the practitioner to apply a stage to a person's response. Once the stage on the TTM has been decided, the level of action will then be appropriate to that stage. This may consist of doing very little (not everyone is going to want to change). As behaviour changes, there may be a need to assess 'stages' at each encounter with the person.

The types of action you may take could include:

- *Pre-contemplation:* providing information, highlighting benefits.
- *Contemplation:* examining ways of overcoming barriers, including access, cost, transport, time or fear.
- *Preparation:* support for any last-minute problems, provide additional advice.
- *Action/Maintenance:* continue to support positive choice made.
- *Relapse:* advice to try again when a person is ready, alongside re-checking the stage a person is in.

Case study 1.8 illustrates an example of the TTM in practice, and how these stages can be used in campaign design.

Case Study 1.8   The stages of change in action – stop, yield and go

Kobetz et al. (2005) utilized the TTM by breaking the cycle into three phases rather than six. Each client was asked two questions.

1   Does she *know* about mammograms?
2   Does she *go* for mammograms?

Traffic-light characters were used to indicate a client's readiness to change their behaviours in relation to mammograms. Susie STOP (Red) represents *pre-contemplation*, Yasmin YIELD (yellow) represents *contemplation* and Greta GO (Green) represents *action*. Susie STOP has knowledge barriers, hence she is in the precontemplation phase. Yasmin YIELD considers going for a mammogram but has access barriers, for example cost or transport. Greta GO understands benefits and uses screening services regularly.

Once women were placed in a stage they receive the appropriate 'action'. Those in the Susie STOP phase were given information about the importance of regular screenings and early detection. Those in the Yasmin YEILD phase had discussions of ways to overcome barriers, were given information about low-cost options and ways to decrease discomfort. Those in the Greta GO phase were commended and reminded of the importance of screening.

CONCLUSION

It is no longer acceptable that health promotion campaigns are planned and implemented on an ad hoc basis and the application of theory to practice in interventions cannot be ignored. In order to promote health successfully and reduce ill health, health promoters should design all interventions using theoretical concepts for successful health promotion campaigns. This chapter has drawn attention to a variety of theoretical models that can be used in full or part to help inform health communication programmes, although there are others that are equally important in health promotion, and that practitioners may prefer to use.

Although theoretical models do not provide a full explanation of every factor in the behaviour change process, they identify potential factors or leverage points that may influence decisions that can help in the targeting and structuring of communication. Critics of theoretical models should continue to debate not what is wrong with these models, but how they can be best used to inform future practice to promote health for all.

Summary

- This chapter has discussed the role and application of theoretical models in health promotion practice.
- Two cognitive models, the theory of planned behaviour and the health belief model, and three stage-step models, the transtheoretical model, perceived behavioural control model and the information–persuasion matrix were described and applied to practice.
- The advantages of using theory were highlighted alongside criticisms of the theoretical approach.
- The use of theory in practice was examined alongside the application of theoretical models to health promotion practice.

ADDITIONAL READING

Theoretical models are discussed in more detail by a variety of authors.

Tones, K and Green, J (2004) *Health promotion: planning and strategies.* Sage, London.

The theory of planned behaviour is explained in more depth in Rutter, D and Quine, L (eds) (2002) *Changing health behaviour.* Open University Press, Buckingham.

Some examples of theory-based campaigns in a US context can be found in Rice, R E and Aktin, C K (eds) (2001) *Public communication campaigns*, 3rd edition. Sage, London.

Social and psychological factors in communication

Nova Corcoran and Sue Corcoran

Learning objectives:

- Examine social and psychological factors that influence health promotion and health communication in a health context.
- Explore ways social and psychological factors can impact on health promotion and the implications of this for communication in health promotion.
- Analyse methods of communicating with different audiences taking into consideration their social and psychological characteristics and utilizing the example of attitudinal change.

Chapter 1 described communication in health as a multi-level transactional process of information exchange in a health-related context. In order for this transactional process to be effective, a number of key factors need to be taken into account when starting the design of a health communication campaign. This chapter will consider 'social' and 'psychological' factors of the target group for effective communication planning. Social factors include variables such as age, gender, ethnicity and education. Psychological factors refer to attitudes, beliefs and values. This chapter will examine each in turn and consider how these factors influence communication. It will also investigate the ways these factors enable effective communication in health, and examine how these factors should be taken into consideration when targeting health promotion interventions. Particular attention will be focussed on strategies employed to change and influence attitudes in health promotion practice.

WHY SOCIAL AND PSYCHOLOGICAL FACTORS?

It is important for a health practitioner to have a clear rationale behind their work. This includes analysis of why a particular topic is being selected for an intervention, why a particular target group is in need of the intervention planned, why the proposed methods have been selected, and identification of an evaluation strategy. Effective health promotion work will assess the need for an intervention before the target group is mapped in detail.

To enable an intervention to fit into the wider health promotion and public health field it is important to first look externally at the planned intervention, before turning thoughts inwards to internal aspects. The external environment refers to the wider environment in which health promotion takes place. Policies, priorities, programmes, political climate, societal influence, rules and regulations will all impact on a choice of health promotion intervention. Any intervention that strives to be effective should therefore take into consideration these factors. Programmes should fit with current philosophy and ideology of policies that already exist at local, national or international level. A good health practitioner will be familiar with the policies and programmes that impact on their work.

Activity 2.1: Policies and practice

An intervention to reduce rates of CHD by increasing physical activity rates in adults would be in line with national UK government recommendations on increasing physical activity from the *Choosing health: making healthy choices easier* document DOH (2004). Internationally this is in line with the WHO's *Global strategy on diet, physical activity and health* (WHO 2004).

1 Think about which policies locally, nationally or internationally impact on your role as a health promoter and the areas that you work in (or are interested in working in) as a health promoter.

Another reason for ensuring that planned interventions fit with current policies and programmes is that priority areas are often more likely to receive funding or resources. Priority areas may be more likely to attract attention of media or other organizations that you want involved in your intervention. Policies are often widely available in libraries and through *information technology (IT)* (for example ◀◀ websites or databases). If the issue you are looking at is not a priority it may have less chance of becoming one, and resources or funding may be less forthcoming. Health practitioners should also stay alert for changing policy and guidance that could have an impact on practice.

Activity 2.2:   Who gets priority?

You are working for a health organization that has received four grant applications for £10,000. Read through these brief descriptions and decide which *one* you will award the £10,000 grant to. (You cannot split your money between others, and the other grants applications will receive nothing). Once you have chosen one application, turn to the back of this textbook and look under the Chapter 2 Activity discussions section for the edited list of *'Choosing health'* (DOH 2004) current priorities.

a   A local sexual health service that specializes in young people has been failing to meet its targets and wants to appoint a new outreach worker. £10,000 would cover an outreach worker's part-time wages for two years.

b   A local project involving two primary schools aims to encourage young people to walk to school. It will cost £10,000 to add a school crossing for peak hours to a busy main road, which runs between one of the most populated areas of town.

c   A local project for single parents wants to develop re-usable 'toy parcels' for those children who have no toys in their home. The funding will be all the money they need to run the programme, as the programme will be self-sustainable.

d   A project to encourage Asian women to attend screening services for breast cancer. The money will be used to enable the service to run at different times of the day, with the involvement of an Asian women's health advocacy worker for one year.

1   Does the one you chose fit into any of the current *Choosing health* priorities?
2   If it does not fit with current priorities, why might you not get the money?

A second consideration when planning interventions is which topic with which group? Interventions have different rationales, and reasons why interventions are being planned are important considerations. These can include:

- A local, national or international priority.
- A high mortality rate or high morbidity rate.
- A gap in a service.
- A problem identified by health practitioners.
- A response to a demand (in a service or group).
- Available resources, skills or practitioners.
- Extra or additional funding.

The decision to choose the intervention in that area will be either a 'reactive' response or a 'proactive' response, or a combination of the two. A reactive decision is something a user group has suggested or a gap in a service, thereby 'reacting' to a problem or demand; for example, a community group formulating a neighbour-hood watch scheme in response to increasing crime rates in that area. A proactive decision is something a health practitioner has decided there is a need for, or that statistics show there is a need for, thus proactively seeking to meet a need or to fill a gap; an example could be the opening of a new stop-smoking service by a health promotion team in response to increasing rates of mortality from tobacco in the local area.

Activity 2.3:   Reactive or proactive?

Which of these is proactive, which is reactive, and which might be both?

1   Providing a free bus service to a local leisure centre, as some community groups have complained of poor bus routes.
2   Allocating money to a local school for a dental project, as it has the highest rate of dental cavities in that community.
3   Raising awareness of HIV on World Aids Day in a local community.
4   Implementing a fitness class in a workplace at lunchtimes after staff indicated that this activity and time-slot would encourage them to take up physical activity.
5   Encouraging self-examination for testicular cancer in male students.

As a health practitioner a balance between the two is important. A campaign that is completely reactive may not be in line with the fundamental aims of health pro-motion/health education. Reactive responses may also not be able to fulfil all the demands made via funding, resources or specialists in that area. An approach that is too proactive may exclude the target group altogether and be taking an authori-tarian 'top-down' approach; as a result your campaign could be ignored by the target group.

THE TARGET GROUP

According to Morrell, 'communication is linked to the social environment in which it is taking place' (2001: 33). From this premise Morrell identifies a variety of social factors which can effect communication, including age, gender, social class, ethnicity, social status, language, power and social relations (such as roles or scripts). Thus, in the wider environment that communication takes place, there are influential factors which impact on the communication process. These are all fac-tors, or traits, that each person has, and will vary between person to person. These factors will influence a variety of processes in communication, including with how, when and where communication is received and how it will be acted upon.

Figure 2.1 illustrates how some of these factors influence a person. In the inner circle are social factors such as age, gender or ethnic group. In the middle circle are psychological factors such as attitudes, *values* or beliefs, and the outer circle contains the wider environment incorporating factors that impact on both social and psychological factors.

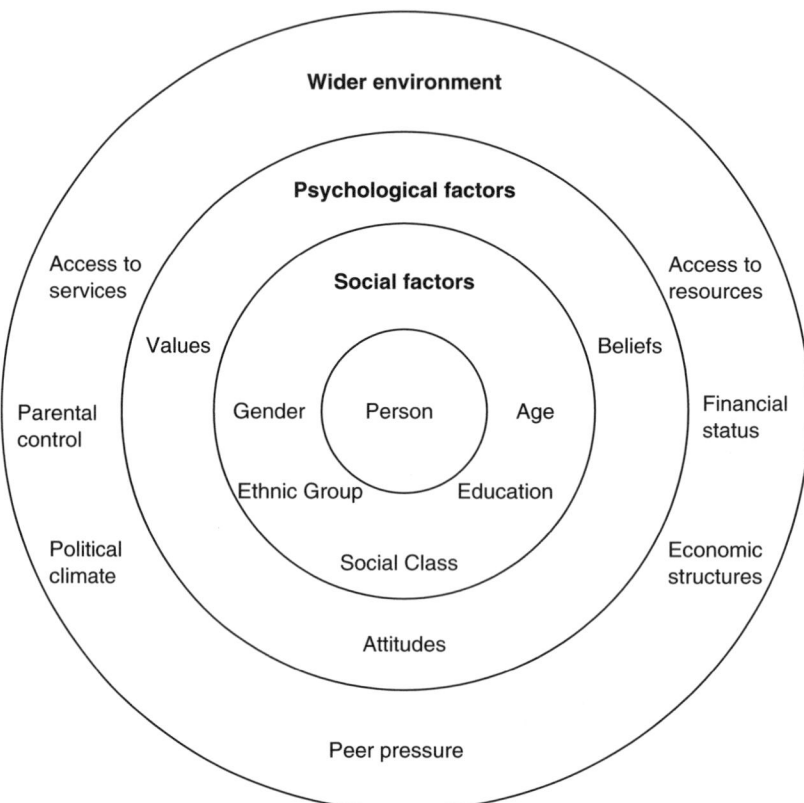

Figure 2.1   Social and psychological factors and the wider environment

As Figure 2.1 suggests, social factors impact on psychological factors and the attitudes, beliefs and values that each person has. This suggests, in the planning stages of health promotion, that these factors will need to be taken into account. For example, social factors can influence how individuals perform protective behaviours, such as regular physical activity. Different groups will perform this behaviour in different ways; young age groups might partake in all physical activity in a school setting, older age groups might use the gym. Social factors also impact on an individual's attitudes, beliefs or values to performing behaviours and thereby need high priority in any proposed health communication project.

Activity 2.4:   Differences in health behaviours

A 17-year-old male will probably not perform the same health-related behaviours as a 17-year-old female. For example, in relation to driving, males are more likely to drug-drive and drink-drive than their female counterparts (Neale et al. 2001) and are also more likely to have an accident on the road (Lancaster and Ward 2002).

1   What different health behaviours might there be between a 25-year-old female and a 60-year-old female?
2   What different health behaviours might there be between a 50-year-old male and a 50-year-old female?

The assumption, based on differences in social factors, is that the more pre-planning that takes these factors into consideration, the more realistic the outcomes of the intervention will be, and the more likely that the target group will be responsive to an intervention.

Although groups can share similar characteristics (for example, age or ethnic group), psychological factors are frequently pertinent to an individual and often internalized so they cannot be seen by others (thus making our 17-year-old in the example above different from other 17-year-olds). Psychological factors include attitudes, beliefs and values and can influence a person's communication and likelihood of adherence or reception to that communication internally. Some groups can share similar attitudes, beliefs or values, but if a mix of social factors is also added, it becomes less likely that all the people in that group will be identical.

THE RELEVANCE OF SOCIAL AND PSYCHOLOGICAL FACTORS TO COMMUNICATION

Individual differences cannot be examined by themselves. Street explains: 'individual difference cannot be examined in isolation of other variables or processes that also account for communicative action' (2002: 201). Robinson and Gilmartin (2002) also indicate that age, gender, socio-economic diversity and ethnic diversity all impact strongly on communication.

Although this textbook will look at each factor in turn, in practice psychological and social factors combine together (as shown in Figure 2.1). Hopman-Rock at al. (2004) provide an examination of determinants of participation in a health exercise and education programme transmitted via television in the Netherlands. They found that higher age (older), female gender, positive intention, knowledge and lower barriers were associated with participation in the health education programme. This example illustrates that links between social and psychological factors both need careful consideration. There are two main ways social and psychological factors should be identified when planning and targeting health communication interventions.

1   Social and psychological factors need to be taken into consideration when *targeting* health promotion interventions. Questions to ask include:

   • Which groups perform (or do not perform) certain behaviours?
   • What are the needs of the target group?
   • What benefits might the target group experience if they perform a behaviour?
   • What barriers do the target group experience to performing a behaviour?

2   Social and psychological factors need to be taken into consideration when *planning* which communication methods to use. Questions to ask include:

   • Which medium will appeal to this group?
   • What messages need to be transmitted to this group?
   • How will messages be framed to appeal to this group?

The more attention that goes into mapping these variables, the more likely the health communication will be relevant, appropriate and well targeted. This strategy is in line with recommendations made by the former *Health Development Agency (HDA)* (2005) in the UK, which suggests targeted and tailored information is imperative for an effective and successful health promotion intervention.

SOCIAL FACTORS OVERVIEW

This section will consider age, sex and gender, socio-economic class and education levels and ethnicity and culture.

Age

The age of the target group influences information preferences for health promotion messages. Factors such as the language or dialect that is used in a health promotion intervention can have an effect on the target group. Different age groups use, understand and interpret language differently.

Activity 2.5:   Differences in communication

1   When communicating a message about good dental hygiene to a 7-year-old and a 50-year-old, what differences might there be between the two?

Different age groups seek health information from different sources. Research shows that television is cited by younger age groups as a health information preference and there were decreasing reports of the use of television as a source of health information with age (Kakai et al. 2003). Kakai et al. also found that newspapers and magazines were perceived as an important source of information in younger age groups, and health professionals were seen as a valuable source of information in older age groups and this importance increased with age. Peterson et al. (2005) found in a physical activity campaign that television was effective in reaching 18–30-year-olds, although it had less impact on intention to exercise than in those who saw the advertisements on billboards and bus wraps. This suggests careful analysis of information preferences that are most likely to lead to action is valuable.

There are also differences in sub-sections of age groups. Austin (1995) split young audiences into subsections, for example 'preschool 0–5' to 'late adolescence 16+' and proposes that credible sources change over time. The 'preschool 0–5' group watch children's television programmes and are influenced by parents. The 'late adolescence 16+' utilize media such as posters, music television and soap operas. A study by Graff et al. (2004) found differences in attitudes to the Internet with lower age groups (17–19) reporting more positive attitudes than older age groups (21–32). Again, this highlights the need to consider the target group in detail, rather than making estimations that everyone in that age range behaves identically.

Age can influence reactions to message content. For example, Henley and Donovan (2003) illustrate that scare tactics in the media have little effect on older females, who respond significantly more to non-threats, whereas older males were seen to respond more to scare tactics. The wording of health promotion messages will also need consideration. How a health product is labelled or packaged has an impact on different audiences. Wardle and Huon (2000) found that children rated a 'healthy labelled' drink as 'less pleasant' and said they would be less likely to ask their parents to buy the drink, illustrating that highlighting health benefits of an activity or behaviour may not be an incentive to younger age groups.

Sex and gender

Sex and gender are important components of the communication process. Sex differences determine the medium and message sought for health communication. Gender, although often the term used to classify men and women, is actually not the biological difference between men and women (sex) but the masculine or feminine *qualities* that a male or female may possess. A study by Kakai et al. (2003) found that females are more likely to obtain their health information from health care professionals and males from newspapers, suggesting a difference in information-seeking preferences. Peterson et al. (2005) postulate that in promoting physical activity to women in the 18–30 age range, television was an effective way of reaching this group. Bessinger et al. (2004) consider multi-media exposure on knowledge and use of condoms in Uganda, and indicate exposure to general media messages regarding sexually transmitted infections (STIs) were more likely to predict a female likelihood of using a condom at the last sexual encounter but not male. Although they additionally propose that men were more responsive to a radio message than women. This highlights differences between channel and content of the message in relation to audience preference and exposure.

Marston (2004) suggests that there are differences between the way men and women communicate and want to be communicated with and that these are often socially determined. Investigation into what is best for the target group needs consideration, and if the target group is mixed, messages and mediums will need to be acceptable and effective with both groups. For example, it will be difficult to foster communication between sexes if topics being covered are traditionally taboo. Sivaram et al. (2005) found in India that spousal communication around the topic of sex and sexual health was minimal, although unmarried men were more likely to discuss sex and sexual health. It might be more appropriate in the first instance to develop interventions that focus on unmarried men's discourse in sexual health, rather than promoting mixed-sex discourse that is more challenging.

Socio-economic class and education levels

Language, medium and location of where an audience accesses health messages can vary depending on social structure or class and education levels. Different social classes use language in different ways, and education levels can be influential in how people respond to health communication. Little educational background may mean difficulties in learning new facts or remembering knowledge (Povlsen et al. 2005). Low education levels may also mean only partial understanding of complex messages. Hussain et al. (1997) found that mother's literacy levels and socio-economic status were important factors for the comprehension of messages about vitamin-A in Bangladesh, with lower literacy levels having less comprehension of messages.

Preference of information source has also been found to be influenced by education levels. O'Malley et al. (1999) found that increasing education levels were associated with more reliance on television as a source of health information. They also found that lower education was associated with reports of not being able to get any health information. Kakai et al. (2003), in work with cancer patients, found that higher education levels were associated with wanting objective, scientific and up-to-date information. Lower education levels were associated with interpersonally communicated information. To add to this, Ribisl et al. (1998) investigated cardiovascular disease risk and found that men with lower education levels obtained fewer health messages from print media and engaged in fewer discussions regarding health matters than those men who had higher education levels.

In groups where socio-economic status is less clear there may be distinctions between the status and power of groups within those societies. Some groups have higher status or more power over members of that group. People can be divided into categories by social traits (Morrell 2001), for example, by sex where authority of men over women is advocated. Alternative groups may be based on age, with elders having more power than younger people, or education, where those who have the most knowledge have the most power. If health communication is trying to access a group that has little power or prestige, it may be difficult to reach those for whom the message is intended.

Ethnicity and culture (see additionally Chapter 3)

It has been acknowledged that individual needs of minority ethnic groups are not always met adequately in the health promotion context. Robinson and Gilmartin (2002), for example, highlight possible problems in communicating health messages including *stereotyping* and typifying people as to how they might behave, ◀◀ such as through racist, discriminatory or prejudicial practice. Other problems cited include miscommunication in language and different meanings of lexical content of words and phrases. Different cultural beliefs can also mean that traditional Western forms of communicating health information are poorly designed (Povlsen et al. 2005) and therefore do not have the desired impact on the target group. Language barriers in particular are important in health promotion work. They can contribute to poor health communication and present a disparity between those who can speak the predominant language and those who cannot. For example, Jacobs et al. (2005) found that women who spoke little or no English in an English-speaking country were less likely to receive screening for breast and cervical cancers, particularly cervical cancer.

Although research is limited, there is evidence to suggest that different ethnic groups may access health information from different sources (O'Malley et al. 1999). Kakai et al. (2003) found differences in health information needs in the three groups they examined. Caucasian patients preferred objective, scientific and updated information obtained through a variety of sources including medical journals, newsletters and the Internet. Japanese patients preferred commercial sources of information gained via television, books and magazines. Non-Japanese Asians and Pacific Islanders preferred person-to-person information sources gained from physicians or their social groups. Although this study examined only three ethnic groups, the assumption is that different groups will have different information preferences, as do different age and gender groups.

SOCIAL FACTORS AND HEALTH PROMOTION PRACTICE

Communication should be designed to take into consideration the range of social factors of the target group. Large-scale mass media campaigns are designed to take into account the social factors of the audience and will have clear age, gender, class and education categories in mind in the design of a campaign.

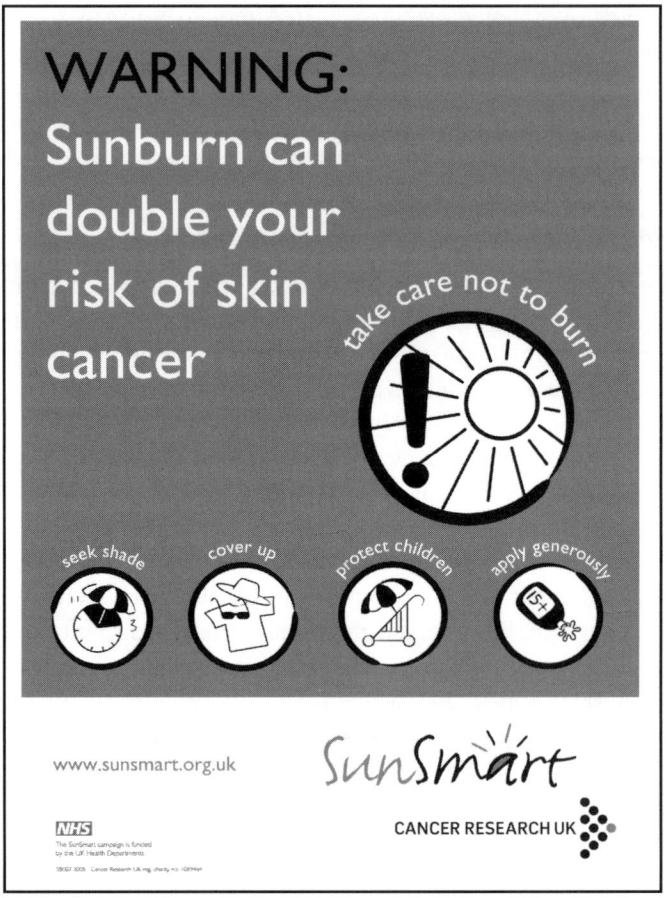

Figure 2.2   SunSmart Cancer Research poster, reproduced by kind permission of Cancer Research © (2006)

Activity 2.6:   Who is the message designed for?

Look at Figure 2.2 SunSmart Cancer Research image. Consider who the poster is designed for under the following headings:

1   What age is the material aimed at?
2   What sex is the material aimed at?
3   What socio-economic status is the material aimed at?
4   What education level is the material aimed at?
5   What ethnicity is the material aimed at?

PSYCHOLOGICAL FACTORS OVERVIEW

Previously, discussion has focussed on social factors, which are externally visible factors. Psychological factors are internal variables which influence a person's decision to perform an action or behaviour. In the case of health these psychological variables are linked to the performance of health promotion or health preventive actions and behaviours. In health promotion the three factors that have received the most attention are attitudes, beliefs and values. An understanding of these factors can assist in the formulation of effective interventions in health promotion. Attitudes have received the most attention and are arguably the most influential of the three factors, thus many health promotion campaigns have aimed to change, influence or challenge attitudes. A number of campaigns based in theoretical models have also sought to examine attitudes, beliefs and values and their role in behaviour change.

Attitudes, beliefs and values can be hard to observe, although a person's beliefs and values often predict an attitude, and this can then be observed by others in the form of behaviour (Morrell 2001). Thus we should be able to observe behaviour and formulate what the attitudes, beliefs and values might be, bearing in mind that psychological factors do not always predict a behavioural outcome and can be unpredictable in nature.

ATTITUDES

'Attitude change has occupied a prominent part in traditional health education' (Tones and Green 2004: 219) and it is often considered to be an important part of health promotion in the move to encouraging individuals to adopt healthy practices. Attitudes occupy a central role in health promotion practice as they are closely linked to beliefs and values. What attitudes are and how they can be changed or influenced has always retained a lively debate.

Attitudes have been defined as relatively stable with consistent tendencies (Naidoo and Wills 2000). This denotes that attitudes can change or can be changed, and also to some extent can be predicted in response to certain situations. What is important is the word 'relatively', meaning that attitudes are not always stable or consistent and therefore do not always correspond to behaviour. It is important to be clear 'about the consequences which can realistically be expected' (Downie et al. 1992) from a programme that seeks to influence or change attitudes. In health this may mean that a smoker who believes tobacco causes premature death and lung cancer may continue to smoke, or a sedentary person who believes exercise will help to loose weight remains sedentary. Because attitudes do not always correspond to behaviour they may conflict with other attitudes or go against certain social or group norms.

Activity 2.7:   Attitudes and complexity

A 14-year-old 5-a-day smoker may have a mixture of attitudes to cigarette smoking. On the one hand they may express positive attitudes to smoking, for example, 'I think smoking makes me look older' or 'All my friends do it, it's a social thing we do

(Continued)

together'. On the other hand they may also express negative attitudes to smoking, for example, 'My parents don't like smoking and they don't know I smoke' or 'I don't like the smell of smoke'.

Remembering that attitudes can be contradictory and complex, and using the example above to help you, read the following sentences and list what 'attitudes' the people might have to the below examples:

1   A 35-year-old regular jogger to going out running in the rain.
2   A 29-year-old who has just been cleared of a suspected melanoma to tanning in the sunshine.
3   A 50-year-old non-seatbelt wearer to driving without a seatbelt.

Attitudes are made up of three aspects: cognitive, affective and conative:

- *Cognitive*: the cognitive aspect relates to the individual's evaluation of that attitude based on the knowledge, facts or information they have. For example, a person may know that taking anti-malaria tablets can prevent malaria in a high-risk zone, but they may also know other people who don't take anti-malaria tablets and have not contracted malaria. The cognitive aspect is the 'weighing-up' process of all the knowledge held about that behaviour or action.
- *Affective*: the affective aspect is the part that includes likes and dislikes, feelings or emotions. For example, a person may want to cut down their fatty food intake, but enjoys the taste of fast food and likes the fact that it is convenient, thereby involving no preparation. The person may dislike the fact that they have put on some weight recently associated with their fast-food intake. The affective aspect is the 'weighing-up' process of likes and dislikes of the behaviour.
- *Conative*: the conative aspect is the behavioural intention towards the 'attitude' object; for example, a person may *intend* to avoid the gym, or a person may *intend* to wear a seatbelt.

Research has found a relationship between positive and negative attitudes to performing health behaviours. Pötsönen and Kontula (1999) examined attitudes to condoms among 15-year-old adolescents. They found that adolescents were knowledgeable about condom use and prevention, but that attitudes of adolescents who did not use any contraceptive methods were more negative to purchasing condoms than those who used contraceptive methods. This suggests that although adolescents have knowledge about the preventive role of a condom, different attitudes influence the actual use of condoms.

A similar finding is reported by Maziak et al. (2004), who examined attitudes and beliefs to *narghile* smoking (smoking tobacco through a water pipe) in a student population. They found that attitudes and beliefs to *narghile* use varied with gender and current smoking status. Positive attitudes to smoking, for example, the attitude that 'smoking was a way of socializing and spending leisure time', were associated with those that smoked. Non-smokers cited more negative attitudes to smoking, including 'pollution' and 'smoke as a nuisance'. Interestingly, however, more smokers than non-smokers said what they disliked the most were damaging health effects, citing main health risks including cancer and respiratory disease, suggesting a contradiction in attitudes. Case Study 2.1 suggests that it is possible to change attitudes via a variety of strategies.

Case Study 2.1   HIV/AIDS intervention in Nigeria

Ezedinachi et al. (2002) designed an intervention that targeted health workers to try to change attitudes and knowledge in Nigeria of HIV/AIDS. They used a mixture of lectures, role play, seminars, group discussion and audiovisual material over two days, and there was a strong focus on discrimination and human rights issues to foster attitude change. Results from this study indicate a decrease in fear levels from HIV and increased sympathy and professional responsibility. They also found that there was increased belief in perceived skills, for example, the ability to provide care and willingness to teach others.

BELIEFS

A belief is a cognitive construct (Tones and Green 2004) and is the information that a person has about an object or action (Naidoo and Wills 2000). An individual's behaviour is linked to their beliefs. Beliefs cannot be directly observed, but are often inferred based on a person's behaviour (Robinson 2004). The individual's personal experiences inform the core beliefs that a person holds.

In health promotion the prediction is that if someone believes something then they will perform that behaviour. For example, if a person believes that wearing reflective clothing when running at night will means cars can see them, they will wear reflective clothing. A person who believes eating fresh fruit and vegetables will decrease the risks of bowel cancer will eat fresh fruit and vegetables. Of course, in reality it is not as simple and beliefs do not always predict or result in the performance of that behaviour. For example, Byrd et al. (2004) found that young Hispanic women, despite believing that they were susceptible to cervical cancer and that screening was beneficial, still had a low rate of compliance to cervical screening. This illustrates that beliefs in the risks of cervical cancer do not necessarily translate into preventive behaviours.

VALUES

Values can influence attitudes by determining the importance attached to them, they 'energise' attitudes and underpin behaviour (Tones and Green 2004). Values are usually acquired through the social world. Friends, family, society, employment or religion are all linked to values and can therefore be linked to personal or cultural values. These values can be explicit or implicit:

- *Explicit values* are those value judgements that are made and can be seen, for example, verbally discriminating against the opposite sex in a social setting.
- *Implicit values* are values that are inferred by non-verbal behaviours, for example, ignoring all members of the opposite sex in a social setting and only talking to those of the same sex.

In relation to health, the role of values suggests that a person puts a 'value' on an object or behaviour. If they regard an object or behaviour highly, for example a cigarette, then they may be more likely to smoke. If they do not value cigarettes highly they are more likely to not smoke. A person will do the same with health promotion and preventative behaviours. If a person values an aspect of health highly, such as mobility or weight loss, they are more likely to attach high importance to activities that seek to achieve those behaviours, such as regular physical activity.

PREDICTING ATTITUDES, BELIEFS AND VALUES IN PRACTICE

When designing health promotion interventions, part of the design process should be to identify attitudes, beliefs and values in the target group, particularly when the use of a theoretical model (such as those in Chapter 1) includes these variables in the behaviour change process. Although this would usually be done in consultation with the target audience, it is possible (although not always advisable) to predict possible attitudes, beliefs and values of a target group.

Activity 2.8:   Attitudes, values and beliefs

List what **attitudes**, **values**, and **beliefs** a person may have to the behaviour below – remembering that values and beliefs may change this. For example:
A young mother who wants to breastfeed her baby and has friends who all bottle-feed their babies. What is her attitude to breastfeeding.
Attitudes: *positive attitude to breastfeeding (based on beliefs and values); positive attitude to doing what her friends do (i.e. bottlefeeding).*
Beliefs: *breastfeeding is a positive thing to ensure the health of the baby; breastfeeding will help the mother to bond with the new baby.*
Values: *may rate health of baby highly, may rate breastfeeding highly.*
Outcome: *Unless strongly influenced by peer pressure and providing the environment is supportive, the young mother is probably more likely to breastfeed her baby.*

Look at the example of the builder below and list:

1   What attitudes he could have.
2   What beliefs he may have.
3   What values he may have.

A builder who works with hazardous substances as part of his daily work. What is his attitude to respiratory and skin problems?

4   Based on the assumptions made about attitudes, beliefs and values, do you think the builder will continue to work with hazardous substances?

Once attitudes, beliefs and values alongside potential outcomes have been identified, interventions can then be chosen to manipulate, influence, or modify these in order to illicit a change in these factors.

STRATEGIES FOR CHANGING ATTITUDES AND BEHAVIOURS

There are a variety of strategies that have been found to influence and change attitudes. These include changing legislation, teaching skills and challenging existing attitudes through a variety of methods such as *peer education*. Kelman (1961) ◀◀ divides these strategies into two areas: **persuasive communication** and *coercive* ◀◀ *communication*:

- **Persuasive communication** aims to encourage individuals to adopt and internalize attitudes, but to do this communication has to be transactional and response dependent (Cassell et al. 1998). A transactional flow of information needs to take place where the receiver accesses information and then via these transactions is able to act upon that information. 'Response dependent' refers to the 'attention to, adoption of, and elaboration of' (Cassell et al. 1998) the message in question. If the person is not responsive to the message, the message cannot 'persuade'. This transaction and response-dependent process is more likely to take place with information that has an interactive element, and thus involves the receiver in an 'active' transaction of information.
- **Coercive communication** can affect behaviour change more directly and immediately, but usually relies on an authority figure to reinforce behaviour. Policies, rules, legislation or laws that stop people performing behaviours are examples of coercive communication. Legislation can restrict health-damaging behaviours and punish those who continue to perform those behaviours, thus changing society's attitudes towards them. Policies introduced to change behaviour are often accompanied with a change in attitudes. In the UK, for example, the majority of the population will have negative attitudes towards those who do not wear a seatbelt, smoke on public transport or drive above speed limits in residential areas as these behaviours put the health of others at risk. The majority of the population do not engage in these activities accordingly. Those that do, and are found to be doing so, are punished (for example by a fine). Yet the introduction of speed limits in residential areas, no smoking on public transport and the introduction of seat-belt wearing are regulations that have been in existence in the UK only during the last few decades.

Problems arise when policies cannot be enforced effectively or provide little incentive for behavioural change. The new move to ban smoking in public places in the UK means that people's smoking behaviour has had to change in public spaces – although even these laws need public support and appropriate mechanisms in place. Banning all fast food in order to decrease the rates of CHD, for example, would simply not work. Consumer demand for fast food, notions of 'free choice', powerful companies promoting fast food and no alternatives for the provision of healthy food outlets, among other factors, make this a difficult thing to achieve. Environmental changes that accompany legislation are also important. Legislation that stipulates no littering is difficult if there are no litter bins. Despite best intentions, not all policies will be effectively enforced or elicit any attitude change, particularly when people perceive no benefit to themselves.

Changing attitudes is one of the hardest aims of health promotion. According to Downie et al. (1992), attitudes can be changed in two main ways:

1   *The provision of information* via a number of mechanisms, including mass media, IT, person-to-person and group communication. This is the most commonly applied strategy.
2   *Encouraging people to behave in a manner that is inconsistent to their current beliefs.* It is suggested that this could be by direct exposure to different behaviours. This could include role-play, simulation or observation, or by changing the pros/cons or costs/benefits of a behaviour through legislation or policy. Ewles and Simnett (2003) add to this list and also include that methods appropriate to this aim include group work, skills training such as decision-making skills, simulation, *role play* or *gaming*, and assertiveness training.

The first of these strategies (provision of information) sees the information process as one of 'giving' information. This may be passive: the mass media may transmit one homogenous message to a large group, or a more active process via a one-to-one communication, allowing the receiver to ask questions. The second process (encouraging people to act inconsistently) engages the receiver via a range of interactions and adopts a more active approach that could involve assertiveness skills, practical skills or direct experiences of the attitude. Each of these will be considered in turn.

CHANGING ATTITUDES THROUGH INFORMATION GIVING

Changing attitudes through information is a more commonly adopted strategy, given that it can be cost and resource effective. There are a number of factors that should be taken into consideration in message planning and design to make it more likely to illicit attitudinal change. Communication to change attitudes involves 'not only audience perception and interpretation of the message, but also perception of the sources intentions and characteristics' (Tones and Green 2004: 221). These can be divided into three sections: the communicator, the communication and the audience. Each should be taken into account when planning health promotion interventions that seek to change attitudes through information giving.

*   **The communicator** should have prestige and credibility over the proposed target group, alongside sharing similar characteristics. Downie at al. (1992) also note that the more people that like a communicator, the more likely people will pay attention to, and accept, the message, especially if the communicator has similarities with the target audience. The use of opinion leaders in a community group may be helpful for getting a message across, particularly where there are hard-to-access groups.
*   **The communication** messages need to be relevant to the target group at that time. This is more likely to be achieved if social factors are taken into consideration and information is tailored to these, alongside the use of theoretical models. These can help predict attitudes, beliefs or behaviours of individuals that influence communication. Some messages may never reach their intended target as they are too complex, inappropriate or directly challenge beliefs or values. Messages should be simple, and memorable campaigns often have simple messages (see Case Study 4.5). They are also more likely to be responded to if they are positive, rather than negative. Remember, health promotion aims to empower individuals to make healthy choices,

rather than scaremongering people into adhering to a message. The use of 'fear appeals' is considered in Chapter 4. New ways of communicating messages offer ways to engage with different message mediums; for example, there is a rise in the use of art and drama for health promotion, which may be one way of using 'novel' information to promote health (see the end of this chapter). The rising popularity in IT applications such as the Internet may also provide new ways for information to be transmitted (see Chapter 5).

- **The audience** will have had their social and psychological factors early on in a good communication. However, despite all the careful planning, remember that not everyone will listen to and act upon messages, no matter how well designed. An individual may not be ready to receive information or act upon the message due to lack of skills, comprehension, interest or other social factors. The more that a health practitioner knows about the audience before sending the message, the better prepared they will be for audience responses. Although attitudes, values and beliefs, along with current behaviours, will affect audience response to a message, wider societal, political and environmental factors may seal the final decision.

CHANGING ATTITUDES THROUGH BEHAVIOUR

Changing attitudes through behaviour change involves different methods from the traditional educational and information-giving approaches and is less widely used. This is partly due to cost, expertise and resource implications and can be more difficult to design, reaching a smaller number of people and sometimes requiring specialist practitioners. As Downie at al. (1992) write, you cannot paint people's skin colour to make them experience racist reactions or subject people to a nuclear winter to change attitudes to nuclear weaponry, therefore you need to utilize techniques that can imitate these scenarios. Working in small groups or with individuals face-to-face may be utilized via role play, experimental learning, skill teaching or other interactive methods of learning.

Role play and experimental learning usually involve participants taking on the role of a different person in a specified setting and acting out the 'part' that person might play, either by following a script or by improvization. For example, children might be encouraged to practice refusal skills to offers of an illegal drug or cigarettes; publicans might be encouraged to practice skills that could be used to diffuse violent incidents in pubs, or office workers might practice resuscitation techniques. One of the main purposes of role play is that people 'act' what should happen in order to then translate this into the real setting when it occurs. Role play can also be performed to groups (for example, two people 'acting' the part of a patient and health practitioner), which may enable people to 'copy' these skills into their own practice. Experimental learning may go one step further and put people into different situations, for example, driving simulators for learner drivers giving practice that can be translated into a real situation.

Teaching skills is another way to enable an attitude change. This can be done in a variety of ways. A 'mock' incident, for example, with railway station staff could give a scenario of what might happen if there was a person taken ill on a train. Or what would happen if there was a spillage of a dangerous substance? Workers in the organization practice what might happen should this incident take place, and challenges attitudes such as 'It's not my responsibility' or 'It's nothing to do with me' in the event of the incident happening. Other skills might include training a practitioner how to calculate alcohol units to counteract thoughts of 'I don't know how to calculate units, so I don't ask questions about alcohol', or teaching a low-fat cooking class to counteract opinions of 'we don't eat healthily as we don't know how to cook different foods'. These may all serve to challenge attitudes towards those healthy (or unhealthy) behaviours.

Case Study 2.2   MIND promoting positive attitudes to mental distress

MIND is a national UK charity group who promote and support positive mental health and challenge negative attitudes or perceptions around mental distress. Some of their work has focussed on promoting positive attitudes to mental distress. They found the following ways have been shown to promote, facilitate or influence positive attitudes to mental distress.

1. *Raising awareness*
Stigma and prejudice against people with mental health problems are reduced when the general public is better informed.
2. *Person-to-person approaches*
A one-to-one or personal contact approach may be the most successful approach to public education. People may be less prejudiced if they know someone with a mental health problem, especially when people are trusted (for example, a role model) or when key public figures talk openly about mental health.
3. *Education*
Education with teenage groups around mental health issues has been found to change perspectives towards mental health issues. Groups showed more sympathy and *empathy* towards people experiencing mental health problems.
4. *Challenging existing attitudes*
Challenging aspects of the social world, such as language or media representations, may be one way to challenge existing attitudes. One suggestion is to use positive alternatives to the negative language used to describe 'mental distress'. The act of thinking about non-discriminatory terms may enable people to reconsider some of the ideas and images behind our language. Another suggestion is to challenge media stereotypes and representations of mental health users as scary, unpredictable or violent.
5. *Policy changes*
Creation of policy or challenges to existing policies might enable mechanisms that discriminate against mental health users to be removed. These include promoting inclusively mental health service users into community settings.
(MIND 2006)

What is interesting about the MIND case study is that they have used a combination of methods to achieve positive attitudes, suggesting that one method alone is not enough to influence attitudes on a large scale. The move to incorporate a second aim (policy changes) is shown to be an important part of changing attitudes also, alongside continual dialogue around mental health issues in society.

Activity 2.9:   Campaigns to encourage positive attitudes

You are designing a campaign with the aim of encouraging positive attitudes to one of the following: breastfeeding, sensible drinking or recycling, in a small village setting (20,000 residents). Your budget is £2,000.

1   Choose one group in the community to work with and identify the social factors of your proposed target group (choose a group in the community to aim your campaign at).
2   Give an example of someone you might use to 'front' your campaign who has prestige, credibility or similar characteristics to your target group.
3   Remembering that the message should be relevant, positive and simple, formulate a slogan for your campaign.
4   Identify a) what methods you will use in your campaign to try to *encourage positive attitudes*, and b) the setting(s) that you will use.

IMPLICATIONS FOR PRACTICE

There are a variety of aspects to remember in relation to social and psychological factors when designing health promotion campaigns. First, you need to know everything you can that is relevant about your target audience. Map out their social and psychological factors in relation to age, gender, social group, education levels alongside attitudes, beliefs, values and other variables that might be important to your campaign. Your chosen theoretical model may give you some ideas about additional variables, for example perceived behavioural control, subjective norm or benefits and barriers. Ask the target group what information preference they have. Research is limited in this area that can be widely applied to different groups, and with the growth of new technologies (for example, the Internet or mobile phones) preferences for information will change.

Collaborate with representatives from the population in the design of materials. Include the target group in the design of the programme, as they will be able to identify important factors that are essential in health behaviours. Engage key organizations and groups that the target group utilizes or works closely with, and work with gate-keepers or key opinion leaders of different groups; for example, consider the use of wider resources for some groups, such as interpreters for different language groups or the use of youth workers for young people.

When working with different ethnic or cultural groups and lower education levels, educational materials should be adapted to different needs. Consider different ways of imparting information to these groups (see Chapters 4 and 5). Develop, design and distribute accurate information in a culturally sensitive and appropriate way.

Finally, choose your theoretical model and methods carefully. Different theoretical models emphasize areas that might be more relevant to your target group, setting or behaviour. You will also need to select your method according to what you are trying to achieve. One method will not suit all.

CONCLUSION

Current research has under-utilized the role of the target group in the development and design of communication strategies to the detriment of these campaigns, particularly in non-Western populations and hard-to-reach groups. Future research should also consider sub-populations in groups.

A good health communication strategy will have a rationale that is based on a clearly identified target group in terms of both social and psychological factors. Health promotion should plan, implement and evaluate information in a way that allows the desired audience to take in information, digest this and then implement this immediately or at a later date as appropriate. By identifying the social and psychological factors of a group and matching their preferences to information, the outcome is more likely to be relevant, achievable and successful.

Summary

- This chapter has examined the role of the target group in health promotion communication design.
- Identification of factors external to the target group including social and environmental factors have been explored.
- The social factors of age, sex, ethnic group and class, alongside the psychological factors of attitudes, beliefs and values have been examined and their links to the target group demonstrated.
- The role of persuasive and coercive communication has been highlighted alongside strategies for changing attitudes with particular reference to information giving and teaching skills.

ADDITIONAL READING

Psychological and social factors are covered in a range of chapters in Rice, R E and Aktin, C K (eds) (2001) *Public communication campaigns,* 3rd edition: Sage, California.

Ellis, R B, Gates, R J and Kenworthy, N (2001) *Interpersonal communication in nursing: theory and practice.* Churchill Livingstone, London. Chapters 2 and 3 cover social and psychological factors, although from a nursing perspective this is still of use to the health promoter.

Note the journal *Health Education* (2005), Vol. 5, available at www.emeraldinsight.com has a whole issue dedicated to art/drama and health promotion.

Reaching unreachable groups and crossing cultural barriers in communicating health promotion

Barbara Goodfellow and Calvin Moorley

Learning objectives:

- Explain the cultural barriers that exist in relation to communication in health settings and consider ways in which these might be overcome.
- Identify the issues around communicating in health settings with different cultural groups, people living with disabilities and older people and consider ways in which these might be overcome.
- Identify the barriers to communicating health to different cultural groups, people living with disabilities and older people and the implications for practice.

The term 'hard to reach groups' may be used to describe a wide range of individuals and groups of people and may in itself be contested. The term might infer blame and lead in turn to prejudice or discrimination. Nevertheless, it is currently recognized that in the UK there are many sections of our society who are, or feel themselves to be, living on the margins of the mainstream. Politically this status has been recognized and the term 'socially excluded' has been applied to these and many other groups to whom the following discussion is relevant (Kane and Kirby 2002). The specific groups that have been selected for discussion in this chapter are: people from ethnic minority cultures, people living with long-term disability and older people. Issues or difficulties around communication and health are common to them all. What is clear is that in order to deliver, develop or design health care of the best possible standard to these, often high-need groups, good communication between them and the service providers is essential.

Activity 3.1:   Defining hard-to-reach groups

1   Identify groups to whom the term 'hard to reach' could be applied.
2   Make a note of these and give the reasons for your choice.

'Core principle 3' of the NHS Plan (DOH 2000a) states that the NHS will shape its services around the individual needs and preferences of individual patients, their families and carers. The NHS of the 21st century must be responsive to the needs of different groups and individuals within society, and challenge discrimination on the grounds of age, gender, ethnicity, religion, disability and sexuality. The NHS will treat patients as individuals, with respect for their dignity. Patients and citizens will have a greater say in the NHS and provision of services will be centred on patients' needs.

CROSSING CULTURAL BARRIERS (SEE CHAPTER 2 FOR ADDITIONAL INFORMATION ON CULTURAL FACTORS)

The concepts of culture and ethnicity

Although no single definition of culture is accepted by social scientists, it is generally agreed that culture is learned, shared and transmitted from one generation to another. Culture is reflected in a group's values, norms, practices, system of meaning (including language and communication) and way of life. The concept of ethnicity is more problematic but is usually used to denote groups of people who share similar histories which give them a distinct identity (Robinson 2002).

Activity 3.2:   Cultural identity

1   Consider what you think of as your cultural identity.
2   How do you think it impacts (or could impact) on you as a health practitioner in your communication and interaction with others?

Distribution and needs of different groups

The latest census recorded that the majority of the UK population in 2001 were white (92.1 per cent) (ONS 2001). The remaining 4.6 million (or 7.9 per cent) belonged to other ethnic groups. Indians were the largest of these groups, followed by Pakistanis, those of mixed ethnic background, Black Caribbeans, Black Africans and Bangladeshis (ONS 2001). The same data shows that people from minority groups were more likely than white people to live in low-income households. As well as differences in self-assessed general health, men and women varied in their likelihood of having specific diseases. One area where this was particularly marked was in the prevalence of self-reported diabetes. Such findings further confirm the importance of addressing communication between health care providers and minority health care users, especially those who lack fluency in English.

Strategies for enhancing cultural awareness

Kreuter et al. (2002) suggest how health programmes and health promotion programmes in particular might make explicit attempts to develop culturally appropriate strategies to meet the needs of special populations. The authors state that health professionals must be able to identify and describe cultures within a given population and understand how each relates to health beliefs and actions. One of the strategies put forward is that of culturally tailored communication, which can be described as any combination of information or change strategy intended to reach one particular person. This can be contrasted with targeting, which is directed towards groups rather individuals. There is clearly a paradox here in that culture is a shared group characteristic, so if something is not shared can it be cultural? Kreuter et al. (2002) argue that individuals within a cultural group can hold varying degrees of certain cultural beliefs.

To illustrate their contention the authors give the example of a project, 'Cultural tailoring for cancer prevention in black women' (Kreuter et al. 1998), that among other things aimed to increase mammography take-up in African American women by tailoring behaviour change messages in a health magazine. The population was defined in terms of demographic and geographic characteristics that were deemed important on the basis of epidemiological cancer risk data. In addition, four potentially important cultural characteristics of the group were identified: religiosity, collectivism, racial pride and perception of time. These were selected as important for a number of reasons, including that they have been demonstrated to be associated with health-related beliefs or practices, they are measurable and they are sufficiently variable in this population to justify tailoring messages based on individual differences.

Case Study 3.1   Trachoma control programmes and cultural differences

The SAFE strategy for trachoma control was evaluated in eight countries worldwide. SAFE is an acronym for the action that is needed to implement a trachoma control strategy:

S – **S**trategy explaining the disease process and need for trichiasis surgery
A – Mass **A**ntibiotic distribution and acceptance of antibiotics
F – **F**acial cleanliness/hygiene promotion
E – **E**nvironmental changes, such as building and using latrines.

Evaluation of the programmes in these eight countries found that different methods were used in different countries to promote similar SAFE messages. Community meetings were seen as a good place to discuss trachoma, and were conducted in a variety of church, mosque, club or society settings. Where local cultural norms were ignored or where providers failed to approach communities in an appropriate manner, there was some resistance to the programme.

The SAFE message was transmitted via different settings in different countries, including schools-based programmes, mass media messages from different mediums (television, radio) and in different formats including songs and drama. Health centres and clinics and one-to-one work were also found effective in some locations. Locally based communicators were also seen as important as they are known to their peer groups.

(Zondervan et al. 2004)

COMMUNICATING ACROSS CULTURAL BARRIERS – PROCESS AND STRUCTURAL BARRIERS

There is a growing realization of the extent of cultural and language variation among ethnic minority users of health and social services. Despite policy initiatives, empirical studies provide evidence that on an individual face-to-face level the communication needs of ethnic minority groups are not always being effectively met. A combination of barriers has been suggested and often fall into one of two categories: process barriers or structural barriers (see Chapter 2 for more information on barriers).

PROCESS BARRIERS

Process barriers may arise in many situations. In the nursing profession, for example, communication difficulties in caring for people from ethnic minority groups, especially those not fluent in English, may be seen as obstacles to the provision of holistic care and the development of a therapeutic relationship. An ethnographic study by Gerrish (2000) aimed to examine how policy directives concerning the provision of individualized care were modified in their transformation into district nursing practice and what this meant for the care provided to patients from different ethnic backgrounds. Gerrish identified six principles underpinning the philosophy of individualised care expounded by the nurses:

1   Respecting individuality.
2   Holistic care.
3   Focussing on nursing needs.
4   Promoting independence.
5   Partnership and negotiation of care.
▶▶   6   *Equity* and fairness.

Gerrrish (2000) highlights the importance of how these principles are then modified and transformed into practice in the context of policy directives on care delivery and factors outside the nurses' control. Although health promotion work is not always carried out in a nursing-related context, the principle issues are similar in other communication contexts. In health promotion work, these six principles are important, and while not all obvious to large-scale communication efforts, they should be basic principles underlying work with these groups.

Activity 3.3:   Application of six principles of care

Re-read the six principles listed by Gerrish (2000) above.

1   Can you identify what factors might inhibit their transformation into practice into health promotion work in a multi-ethnic society?

There are a number of other barriers to health promotion. For example, in research around female groups, it has been proposed that non-English speaking women may not receive adequate maternity care unless their needs are met via interpreters or advocates (Rowe and Garcia 2003). Jacobs et al. (2005) also found that women who spoke little or no English in an English-speaking country were less likely to receive screening for breast and cervical cancers, particularly cervical cancer. In a health promotion context this may mean the provision of preventative service, or preventative messages, are unable to be transmitted unless adequate alternatives are sought.

Another instance of a process barrier to communication is cited by Vydelingum (2000), who studied a small number of hospital patients and carers in a mixed ethnic minority group. This study found that language barriers and communication difficulties which accompanied this led to feelings of extreme isolation. Vydelingum observed that these communication difficulties were exacerbated by other factors, including:

- lack of positive action on the part of the nurses in providing resources to aid effective communication, and
- that nurses were perceived as too busy to respond to patients' needs in relation to diagnosis, medication and discharge.

Activity 3.4: Overcoming barriers

1 Without adding to the workload of the nurse, and without spending any additional finances, what could you as a health promoter suggest could be done to try to remedy the two factors highlighted by Vydelingum (2000)?

Another factor which might also hinder good communication is the application of caring models in which there is a high expectation of patient involvement which may not be fully appreciated by the patient or their family and would not be the norm in their culture. Stereotyping may also further compound poor communication.

STRUCTURAL BARRIERS

At a time when a major thrust of the modernisation agenda of the NHS (DOH 2000) is the involvement and empowerment of service users, it is vital that minority ethnic groups should not be excluded from this process due to communication barriers limiting their control over care options (DOH 2000). Evidence, however, still suggests that these structural barriers are still in place. Robinson (2002) suggests a number of areas that need to be considered in relation to the way in which organizational aspects undermine the quality of communication and care. He states: 'in the area of assessment of minority ethnic user needs by community consultation, gathering and use of information about individual patients' communication needs, bilingual support, practitioner education, and provision of material resources, organizational shortcomings have been demonstrated' (Robinson 2002: 15).

Case Study 3.2 Black and Afro Caribbean groups and mental health

A well-documented example illustrating how disadvantage in everyday life may inhibit the ability of some groups and individuals ethnic minority groups have introduced user involvement with diagnosis, care and treatment by mental health services.

Baker and Macpherson (2000) found that black and Afro Caribbean people are more likely to:

- Be diagnosed with schizophrenia.
- Receive physical treatment when in care.
- Not receive counselling or psychotherapy or see black counsellors.
- Be regarded as violent, located in locked wards and have longer stays in medium secure care.
- Receive higher doses of medication.
- Find their way into hospital via the police, compulsory admission under the Mental Health Act or from prison.
- Overall, black people have poorer outcomes after care.

(Wallcraft 2003; Fernando 2003)

Activity 3.5: Challenging the present

1   Consider the list in Case Study 3.2 and think about how many items on this list involve communication between the service user and service provider.
2   If you were working with a black or Afro Caribbean group in the community, how might you try to reduce any of these variables via health promotion work?

Reasons given to explain why black people and other ethnic minority backgrounds appear to have higher rates of mental illness and a different, often coercive relationship with services includes: racist and prejudiced attitudes on the part of service providers and agencies of the state, such as the police; a lack of cultural sensitivity; more frequent exposure to stressors such as unemployment; and adjusting to a new society.

It is clear that for many aspects of the NHS modernization agenda to work in reality requires a shift in the balance of power, which must be supported by a real culture change in the way services are provided and particularly in the way in which communication takes place between service providers and users from ethnic minority groups.

COMMUNICATION AND PEOPLE LIVING WITH DISABILITIES

It is estimated that there are around 500 million disabled people worldwide, the largest number of whom are to be found in the developing world. However, there is a higher prevalence of disabled people relative to population numbers in the developed world. It is clear that with advances in medicine which prolong life and the demographic changes in the age of the population these numbers will increase. There are many types of disability, including sensory and learning disability. For the purpose of this analysis the emphasis will be on people living with physical disability.

THE CLASSIFICATION AND DEFINITION OF DISABILITY

The classical way to view disability is to see it as a medical problem. It is this approach that is the basis for most current health and social policy, and also that which lies at the centre of much medical treatment aimed at people with disabilities. It is the basis of the World Health Organization's (WHO 1980) International Classification of Impairments, Disabilities and Handicaps (ICIDH), produced in 1980. This approach assumes that impairments are the result of biological or psychological abnormality, and that disabilities are the resulting barriers to activity and handicaps are the disadvantages faced by people with disabilities as a result of this.

Such classification locates 'the problem' with the individual and provides a deficit model of disability where people with disabilities are viewed as powerless objects of policy rather than as citizens. From 1960 onwards large numbers of disabled people felt that traditional politics had failed them and there was a shift in the way they were managed and treated, with an emphasis on user organization and self-reliance with a political rather than a medical orientation. This shift was also underpinned by the adoption of a social rather than a medical model of health. Oliver (1992) contrasted existing notions of disability, which saw disability as a characteristic of the individual, with a view of disability that is largely political.

LABELLING AND STIGMA

Language is critical in shaping our thoughts, beliefs, values and attitudes. Some words by their very nature degrade and diminish people with a disability. The language customarily used to denote disability has been condemnatory, and perhaps the most dangerous use of language in describing a person with a disability has been to dehumanize the individual by labelling the person as the disability. In the past people with disabilities have been stigmatized. 'Labelling' and 'stigma' are terms used to describe negative evaluations of individuals or groups by other individuals or groups. The terms are important for health workers because their ability consciously or unconsciously to apply such labels to people with disabilities reflects the tradition power held by such workers, especially practitioners in the medical profession.

HEALTH PROMOTION – COMMUNICATION AND LANGUAGE

Thompson (2002) observes that health practitioners who are working with disabled people need to recognize the social roots of disability and stigma so that they can avoid:

- allowing negative stereotypes to mar interpersonal interactions;
- reinforcing or exacerbating the social disadvantages associated with disability; and
- disempowering disabled people.

Health practitioners need to be sensitive to the fact that disability acts as a form of social oppression, and practice therefore needs to be geared towards challenging such oppression rather than reinforcing it. The potential of communication and particularly language to reinforce or exacerbate oppression is often not fully recognized. We need to realize that language not only reflects reality but also contributes to creating and maintaining that reality. Language can transmit the dominant ideas that perpetuate inequality and disadvantage for people with disabilities. Figure 3.1 illustrates the notion that discrimination in society is reflected in language, and in turn language reinforces discrimination in society.

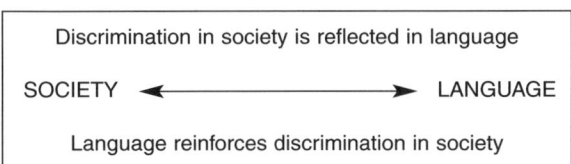

Figure 3.1   The double standard of language and discrimination

HEALTH CARE COMMUNICATION AND DISABILITY

People with disability, and their families, typically have frequent and ongoing communication with a wide variety of health care professionals, depending on the nature and severity of their condition. There is considerable evidence to indicate that patient satisfaction is closely related to the communication skills of health care workers. However, professional communication is an area in which health care provision often does not meet patient needs. Such professional communication might be that with nurses, physiotherapists, occupational therapists and other allied health professionals. Prominent among the health care relationships that have been the subject of previous research is that of the doctor–patient relationship, and while this is recognized as remaining significant there is now increasing attention being drawn to a wider patient experience.

POLICY – THE EXPERT PATIENT

A plan for the establishment of an Expert Patients Programme was announced by the government in thee 1999 Health Strategy White Paper *Saving lives: our healthier nation* (DOH 1999) and later reaffirmed in the NHS Plan (DOH 2000).

An expert patient task force was set up to explore models, review evidence, consider barriers and recommend a programme that would bring together the work done by patient and clinical organizations in developing self-management initiatives in chronic disease. The report *The expert patient: a new approach to chronic illness disease management for the 21st century* was published in 2001 (DOH 2001b). The concept of expert patient now seems firmly embedded in UK health care policy along with the admission that the NHS is not nearly as strong as it could be in meeting the needs of people with disabilities.

Among the models of chronic disease self-management is one developed at Stanford University (Robinson 2002), which recognizes that people with chronic illness deal with broadly similar issues. These include:

- symptom management;
- relaxation;
- problem solving and action planning;
- exercise and nutrition;
- managing fatigue;
- communication; and
- engaging with health professionals.

Thorne et al. (2000) take up the issue of communication and note that although it has become an accepted standard to acknowledge the patient as a full partner in health care decisions, thus replacing traditional authoritative relationships with those based on an emancipatory model, the experiences of people living with chronic illness confirm that this paradigm shift is not yet apparent in many health care relationships. They examine both doctor–patient and nurse–patient communication and conclude that not until all health care professionals have become sufficiently confident in and accepting of the importance of health care relationships as part of chronic illness experience can inappropriate communication be challenged. Figure 3.2 illustrates some aspects of appropriate and inappropriate communication, as adapted from Thorne et al. (2004a). Communication is grouped under the three categories: managing fear, taking charge and crafting a life. In 'managing fear', for example, appropriate information includes pre-planning of appointments and inappropriate includes the dismissal of individual experience. For 'taking charge', appropriate communication is that of the provision of as much information as possible, inappropriate would be providing inaccurate or dated information. For 'crafting a life', appropriate communication would centre round ongoing support and interest, and inappropriate would be when health practitioners give up, become disinterested or withdraw support.

Thorne et al. (2004a) conclude that for the participants in their study, self-care management of chronic disabling conditions is difficult, frustrating and at times overwhelming. It requires persistence, courage and great adjustments. Good health care communication can profoundly influence the patients' ability to live as well as possible and obtain optimal health outcomes.

Coping focus	Appropriate	Inappropriate
Managing fear	• Accurate, appropriate information • Planned appointments	• Withholding information • Dismissing individual experiences
Taking charge	• Providing as much information as possible • Access to health care professionals • Acknowledging limits of medicine	• Inaccurate information • Difficulty in accessing services or health professionals • Belief that medicine will cure all
Crafting a life	• Ongoing support, interest • Ability to explore additional options • Respecting patient as competent and knowledgeable	• Giving up • inflexibility in methods used • Condensation and reprimand

Figure 3.2 Appropriate and inappropriate communication, adapted from Thorne et al. (2004a)

Watson et al. (2006), in an American study, examined the communication processes between parents of children receiving centre-based services for developmental delays and disabilities and the professional providers' services. In this study communication is defined as having both content and relationship dimensions. The core construct that emerged from the grounded-theory approach adopted by the researchers was that of striving for therapeutic relationships within a context of uncertainty. Both parents and health professionals operated in a context of uncertainty regarding the child and his or her development and prospects for the future as well as their expectations of each other. Both parents and providers used strategies of:

- *Balancing* competing needs, competence, the need for intervention, parent and provider roles and the here-and-now and the future.
- *Questioning* used by both parents and providers to get information and evaluate the other person's attitude and knowledge.
- *Reading the cues* including facial expression and body language.
- *Managing the sessions* such as treatment sessions, telephone calls and written communication.
- *Managing uncertainty* coloured all interaction.

The main outcome was that relationships between parents and providers were valued by the extent to which they were seen as therapeutic to parents and child. This study confirms the importance of good communication and interpersonal relationships between the professional, and in this case the parents, contributing to the wellbeing of the parents and the child.

Case Study 3.3   Young disabled peer mentoring and support programme

The Young Disabled People's Peer Mentoring/Peer Support Project as part of The Greater Manchester Coalition of Disabled People (GMCDP) Young Disabled People's Forum developed a range of activities to address needs of young disabled persons over a two-year period. The project was evaluated with the help of both adults and younger disabled people and found that barriers to independence can be reduced by supporting young disabled people in an environment that allows meeting, working and sharing ideas. Young disabled people preferred projects that included a wide range of activities (the projects ranged from social events to campaigning). The evaluation also found that traditional notions of peer education could be too formal and thus less effective. A more flexible model of peer education was seen to be useful in some circumstances.

(Joseph Rowntree Foundation 2003)

Thorne et al. (2004a) explored the communication between people with chronic illness and their professional health care providers in a qualitative secondary analysis of a set of in-depth interviews and focus groups conducted on people with a longstanding multiple sclerosis (MS) experience. Analysis of their accounts illustrates a complex interplay between common features of this particular disease trajectory and the communications that are seen as helpful or unhelpful in living well with the disability arising from this chronic condition. The authors conclude by drawing interpretations for those who care for people with this disease from what might be seen as communication competencies.

DEFINING, PROFILING AND LOCATING OLDER PEOPLE

One of the concerns of health promotion is reaching different groups, and identifying these groups can prove difficult and should be done with great accuracy. The definition of the group labelled as 'older people' has had some differing opinions across the world (Tinker 1997). In the UK the term 'older people' usually refers to those over retirement age. Those concerned with the study of older people have formulated categories of ageing. These are the 'young old' aged between 65–74 years, the 'old old' aged between 75–90 years and the 'very old' over 90 years (Tomassini 2005). The 2001 census confirmed what most people who work with older people thought: that in the UK we have a growing older population. The census (ONS 2001) reports that 336,000 people are aged 90 and over. *Focus on older people* (ONS 2004) reveals that in 2003 there were over 20 million people aged 50 and over resident in the UK. (Chapter 2 also contains links to age and health.)

Ageing is an interesting phenomenon, as being 'old' is often viewed in a biological and social context. The age of an individual is a chronological event, therefore measured in years. More frequently age is measured in abilities, beginning with the young – when a child starts walking or talking – or in other words, through cognitive development. For older adults disabilities are measured in relation to age, mainly in terms of physical and psychological deteriorations. There are three main approaches to defining ageing. First the chronological approach, which looks at the age of the individual in terms of number of years lived. The second approach is based on subjective perception. It takes into account how the individual feels, what their age means to them, and also social meanings of their age. The final approach is linked to social construction, where the social representation of age in institutions (such as hospitals, prisons, universities, colleges) and government departments' ideologies and structural interest determine age. For example, some companies may have different policies on the age of retirement, which may not always be in agreement with national guidelines. Some educational institutions may label their students according to their age, for example students over 21 years in the UK are commonly referred to as 'mature' students. These variations of age are important to bear in mind when designing health promotion work, as a health practitioner will have to consider what sort of 'age' will be used in their work.

The study of ageing and older people falls under the discipline of gerontology and is viewed as a multidisciplinary approach to the study of ageing; rather than a pure science, it draws from the social and physical sciences (Jamieson 2002). This multidisciplinary approach can lead to different emphasis on the health and quality of life of older people. While the physical science may focus on the functional ability of older people, the social science may choose to concentrate on the meaning and value of experiences of ageing. Both are of equal importance to health promoters and planners in meeting the needs of this target group.

Older people, though visible within society, can be difficult to locate, mainly due to the macro (structural and societal) and individual (personal) perspectives. Arber and Ginn (1995) explain that as we age we are influenced by the societal, cultural economic and political context prevailing in our everyday life. This can lead to changes in behaviour and attitude. On a macro level, the values of society concerning older people can lead to this group of older people fulfilling the personal perspective through the disengagement theory process (Cumming and Henry 1961) where the individual, as ageing progresses, withdraws from society and vice versa. Other writers suggest older people should engage more with the activity theory. Havighurst (1963) postulates that in order to age successfully (using Marslow's *hierarchy of need* approach), the older person needs to maintain similar levels of activity as they did in middle age. Closer examination of both theories in the literature shows that they make the same assumptions about all older people. It is this type of generalization that health professionals need to move away from. Policies concerning housing, pensions, allowances and to a greater extent health care can force this group into avenues that are difficult to locate. The macro level influences coupled with the individual perspective can enhance the profile of the invisible population.

HEALTH AND WELLBEING

The ageing process in the UK has been reported as a time of negative decline which exposes individuals to increasing risk of illness and disability. Health is an important concern for older people; it is a period of life where the ability to maintain good health is seen as the key to remaining independent, allowing them to perform normal daily activities. The World Health Organization defines health as a 'completeness of physical, mental and social wellbeing not merely the absence of disease or infirmity' (WHO 1986). This definition can have limitations as we move to a more subjective definition, as for older people health may mean a variety of different things. It may mean the ability to be physically independent, to be able to get from one place to another, which includes driving and the feeling of safety while doing so. It may mean to be financially independent, to be able to make independent choices and not be instructed on what to do but given the freedom of choice, or to be able to have a social network that they can rely on.

Some older people hold the view that being healthy is also being part of a society that values their opinion and their contribution to that society. Alternatively, definitions of health may include good housing, secure buildings, adequate heating, to be able not only to cook a meal but afford to dine out or to live in a safe environment with access to transport facilities (Action for Health 1996; Walker and Maltby 1997; Help Age International 2002). Health is of utmost importance to older people because it reflects their ability to remain independent and disability-free in a period of their life when physical, mental and to a certain level social decline may have adverse effects. The second element of importance is that health professionals and anyone involved in the care of older people acknowledge the subjective definitions of health and build them into the structural/macro concepts of ageing in order to communicate effective health messages to older people.

Case Study 3.4   The Age Concern website

Age Concern, the largest organization in the UK working with and for older people, has a website with information designed specifically for older people. It contains a wealth of information including policy documentation and key issues. It also contains a 'Living room' section with health ageing information including advice around positive mental health, dental care, healthy eating, men's health, giving up smoking and health and wellbeing information for older lesbians, gay men and bisexuals.

To try and facilitate access to their website for those who might have 'accessibility' problems they include a section where information is provided to enable access to the website. This includes advice on increasing font sizes options, changing sound volumes, altering keyboard settings and screen readers problems.

(Age Concern 2006)

COMMUNICATION AND BARRIERS TO WORKING WITH OLDER PEOPLE

The world's population is ageing; in the UK we are now in a low demographic regime (or in other words, a low fertility rate) and a growing larger older population. There are rapid changes to the lives of older people influenced by advanced technology and economic and social developments. Such developments can produce many challenges to providing good quality care to older people. Estimates of the older, longer living population in the UK is steadily increasing. One of the effects of this year-on-year growth is that older people will become the largest consumer group of health and health care provisions. In order to address these needs competently, we need to be able to communicate effectively to the targeted audience on a group and individual level.

As detailed in Chapter 1, communication between individuals and groups is a complex process of 'interaction' whereby there is a sender, a message (through a mode of transmission) and a receiver. In order for communication to occur, the sender must be clear on what message they want to send, choose the appropriate mode of transmission and ensure that the receiver gets the message as it was originally sent or intended.

Activity 3.6:   Communicating with older people

1   Make a list of the different ways you can communicate health messages to older people.
2   Would all these ways of communicating messages be appropriate for all older people? Why/why not?

Knowledge of communication skills is important and can enhance the communication process when communicating health to older people. In order to make full use of verbal and non-verbal communication skills, the health care worker and those concerned with the older person need to have an awareness of the possible barriers to communicating with the group or individual. These barriers can be divided into two categories, arising mainly from the biological (physical) and the psychosocial components of the ageing process.

Due to the changes in physical cell activity (biological), the effect of ageing pathology on the central nervous system can lead to physical decline. Figure 3.3 illustrates the problems and possible solutions to improving communication in groups that may have visual, hearing or speech impairment. Health promotion communication may be more difficult, and may require materials or content to be adapted accordingly.

Figure 3.3 identifies some of the areas that should be considered when communicating messages with an older age group. Many of these may be seen as

Problem	Style of communication	Ways to maximize communication
Visual impairment	Face-to-face/ group	• Direct eye contact • Ensure glasses are clean and the correct pair
	Media-based	• Use large font materials • Use aids such as large print literature, talking books, audio materials • Use the enlarged screen setting for electronic communication
	Other points	• Maintain familiar environment to reduce risk of accidents
Hearing impairment	Face-to-face/ group	• Face the person(s) so that they are able to lip read • Speak slowly and clearly • Use questions and answers to check understanding
	Media-based	• Use communication to enhance the spoken word, e.g. pictures and writing, subtitled audio-visual material, electronic communication (i.e. email)
	Other points	• Eliminate background noise Ensure hearing aids are working and switched on
Speech	Face-to-face/ group	• Speak slowly and clearly using simple sentences • Allow time for the person to respond • Encourage the use of gestures, nodding, blinking, thumbs up etc.
	Media-based	• Choose aids such as pictures, cue cards, written instructions, IT-based programmes (i.e. email, chat rooms)
	Other points	• Observe signs of non-verbal communication (i.e. distress)

Figure 3.3   Ways to overcome visual, speech or hearing difficulties, adapted from Marr and Kershaw (1988)

common sense, for example maintaining eye contact, but these actions can make the difference between comprehension and lack of comprehension of a message. The assistance of additional health professionals such as occupational therapists, speech and language therapists or physiotherapists may be invaluable in your work with different groups within the older age range, especially if the older person is experiencing cognitive impairment. Multidisciplinary working is essential for effective communication with older age groups.

Activity 3.7: 'Stop smoking' materials for those over 70

You are working for a 'stop smoking' service and you have been asked to design some stop smoking information for a group of individuals over 70, some of whom have sight impairments. Based on Figure 3.3:

1 What might you include in the design of your materials?
2 Would you be able to design one resource that would be suitable for everyone?

The other challenges that could be encountered in working with older people include psychosocial barriers. These may exist due to an older individual withdrawing from society (see the disengagement theory discussed earlier), the loss of family or partner, loss of income, moving home to a smaller dwelling, or due to financial difficulties alongside the impact of physical or neurodegenerative disorders. Communication with older people who are cognitively impaired should be undertaken by those who are professionally trained to work with such people, as cognitive impairment can result in memory loss, disorientation, confusion, wandering and problems in recognizing family members and friends.

Activity 3.8: 'Healthy heart' programme design

You are working for a local hospital and you are running a 'Healthy heart' class for the over-sixties. Participants are given a variety of options to try to reduce their risk of coronary heart disease, including light physical activity and healthy eating classes. You want to encourage individuals to attend who have been identified as high risk. These individuals have been sent invitations in the post but so far have not attended, and you suspect this is because they do not want to join a group.

1 What might you do to encourage people to attend?
2 What messages other than 'health' messages could encourage people to attend?
3 What other options could be provided for people who do not want to join a group (apart from meeting people face-to-face)?

OLDER PEOPLES' HEALTH POLICY AND HEALTH PROMOTION

The recent improvements in care and health services for older people in England have been largely influenced by the *National service framework for older people* (DOH 2001c), which advocates eight set standards involving the care of older people (see Figure 3.4).

> **The NSF eight standards for older people are:**
>
> - Rooting out age discrimination
> - Person-centred care
> - Intermediate care
> - General hospital care
> - Stroke
> - Falls
> - Mental health in older people
> - The promotion of health and active life in older people

**Figure 3.4   The National Service Framework for Older People
(DOH 2001c)**

This Framework is the first ever comprehensive strategy to ensure fair, high-quality, integrated health and social care services for older people. It is a 10-year programme of action linking services to support independence and promote good health, specialized services for key conditions and culture change so that all older people and their carers are always treated with respect, dignity and fairness (DOH 2001c).

Activity 3.9:   NSF demonstrated outcomes

The NSF for older people indicates that local health systems have to demonstrate each year improvements in:

- Flu immunisation.
- Smoking cessation.
- Blood-pressure management.

  If you were designing a campaign to increase uptake of services available in one of these three areas:

1   What methods do you think might be appropriate?
2   What key messages might you give that are appropriate for older people?

It is important to acknowledge that this Framework uses the goals of health and social policy to benefit older people. It allows the promotion of health to extend a healthy active life and at the same time trying to compress morbidity. The compression of morbidity is seen as the period of life before death spent in frailty and dependency, (DOH 2001c). The Framework allows health and social care workers to identify emerging problems ahead of crisis and thus reduce long-term dependency. Through the use of this Framework it is easier to anticipate and respond to problems, recognizing the complex interaction of physical, mental and social care factors that may compromise independence and quality of life in older people. This Framework is all-encompassing and enables planning to include global and holistic concepts when designing care for older people. When planning interventions for older people, this policy document is essential in setting targets, specifying target areas and providing guidelines to health promotion work.

Activity 3.10:   A new ambition and mental health

Gains in the health of older people is built upon and embodied in the government's paper *A new ambition for old age* (DOH 2006a). This is the next step in fully implementing the National Service Framework for older people (DOH 2001) within areas where targets have not been achieved, such as intermediate care and mental health needs. The paper has ten programmes under three themes.

You are working for Age Concern, and your remit is to improve the mental health of older people in a rural area:

1   What interventions might you suggest to help improve the mental health of older people?
2   How might the older people access support for mental health problems, given they are in a rural area (transport is limited)?

One of the challenges for health promotion in older people is to identify the opportunities in old age for improving health. To achieve this effectively we need to take account of differences and changes in lifestyle and the impact of cultural and religious beliefs. Cultural and religious beliefs can be accommodated in local health strategies that specifically promote healthy ageing for the selected client group. When planning local health promotion activities for older people it must be acknowledged that older people are not homogenous but are a diverse group, in terms of health and fitness, dependency, socio-economic status, levels of social exclusion and ethnicity. Chapter 2 discusses social and psychological factors of target groups in more detail.

CONCLUSION

As part of a health task force, we need to assess continually how we can reach individuals and groups in order to deliver health promotion. To achieve this goal health practitioners will need to be objective, with a level of sensitivity that will allow them to reach a group that can often be hidden within the wider community. The first step starts with listening. There needs to be greater consultation with groups: different cultural groups, people living with disabilities and older people. These include the people themselves, networks and advocates in order to be able to assess their health promotion needs. Always ask the target group what they want before planning an intervention. The second stage needs to assess current legislation and look at the different ways that these groups can become more inclusive in local policy and health agendas. Finally, the strategies used in health promotion need to reflect the time and place the targeted group lives in.

New technology may go some way towards meeting health needs, for example, the use of computers and mobile phones can be useful in helping older people to better understand health and meet their own health needs. This could include ▶▶ *SMS messaging* or e-mail for GP appointments. Another example can be creating ▶▶ online *chat rooms* about issues identified by target groups, for example, different cultural groups. This can be moderated for and by the target group with the assistance of health professionals, and is a simple way of targeting this group. By allowing people to participate in the setting up of the system, we are using the participatory approach with an emancipatory goal. In reaching these hard-to-reach groups we not only impart health but also learn, and it is this symbiotic relationship that allows us to work in harmony.

Summary

- This chapter has explored the role cultural groups, people living with disabilities and older people in relation to health promotion and health care.
- It has identified issues around communicating with these groups, alongside highlighting barriers to communication with these groups.
- This chapter has explored strategies and solutions to overcoming these barriers to enable health promotion communication in these hard-to-reach groups.

ADDITIONAL READING

There are a number of resources available for additional reading. Textbooks that give you a wide range of views include:

Fernando, S (2003) *Cultural diversity, mental health and psychiatry*. Routledge, London.

Robinson, M (2002) *Communication and health in a multi-ethnic society*. Policy Press, Bristol.

Jamieson, A and Victor, C (2002) *Researching ageing and later life*. Open University Press, Buckingham.

4

Mass media in health communication

Nova Corcoran

Learning objectives:

- Analyse the role of mass media in health promotion programmes and campaigns.
- Explore the design of mass media campaigns utilizing best practice and the principles of social marketing for health promotion.
- Examine current debates in the use of media and exploring the alternative roles of media in health promotion contexts.

The use of mass media in health promotion has been widely employed and continues to be an attractive way to promote health to the wider population. Mass media is most frequently utilized in health promotion to provide information about health issues alongside attempts to promote behaviour change. Mass media is also used to raise awareness of health topics to the wider population alongside promoting societal, political or environmental change. This chapter will examine the role of mass media in health promotion and health education. It will also discuss effective strategies for mass media, including consideration of the limitations. Alternative ways of utilizing the media in health promotion will be explored, including social marketing principles and media advocacy.

WHAT IS MASS MEDIA?

The use of mass media as a tool to promote health has been utilized extensively (Noar 2006). Although practitioners are now more realistic about the outcomes of media use, it remains attractive to health practitioners due to its wide-reaching, appealing, powerful nature alongside its cost effectiveness (Randolf and Viswanath 2004). The mass media has the ability to reach a large number of people simultaneously (Tones and Green 2004), either locally, nationally or internationally. Early beliefs around mass media use centred around mass media's apparent powerful effect on the receiving audience. It was prophesized that whole populations would heed mass media health education messages and adapt their behaviour accordingly. Of course if this were the case societies worldwide would be filled by populations who drink sensibly, do not smoke tobacco, eat reduced-fat diets rich in essential vitamins and minerals and engage in other protective and preventative behaviours. As it became clear that this was not the case, health practitioners have begun to move towards a more realistic concept of mass media use in their work.

Mass media is any type of broadcast, printed or electronic communication medium that is sent to the population at large. For the purpose of this textbook, mass media will be divided into four broad categories: audio-visual broadcast media, audio-visual non-broadcast media, print-based media and electronic media. Figure 4.1 illustrates this division in more detail and provides examples of how these categories are used in health promotion work.

Type of media	Example of media	Ways to use media
Audio-visual broadcast media	Television, radio	News programmes, documentaries, soap-operas, education-entertainment, public service announcements (PSA), advertisements
Audio-visual non-broadcast media	Videos, DVDs, CDs, cassette tapes	Self-help packages, advertisements, documentaries, short features, cartoons
Print media	Newspapers, magazines, leaflets, pamphlets, booklets, journals, books, photo-comics, billboards, *bus-wraps*	News items, magazine features, advertisements, stories, reports, cartoons, story-boards
Electronic media	Internet, CD-ROMs, mobile phones, computer packages, touch-screen kiosks	Websites, self-help packages, information packages, text messaging

Figure 4.1   The four categories of mass media

Audio visual broadcast media includes television and radio. This could be used in the creation of news items, the advertisement of health products, public health service announcements, or even in soap-opera and dramas. Audio-visual non-broadcast media refers to media that is not broadcast over a recognized channel. This could include videos or DVDs, and could be used to give information via a short feature or programme, a short documentary, or in the provision of self-help information. Print-based media (often the most widely used in health promotion) includes newspapers, magazines, leaflets and billboards. Print media can be used for information giving via leaflets, coverage of a health topic in a news item, short stories, cartoons or magazine features. Electronic media (discussed in depth in Chapter 5) includes the Internet, CD-ROMs, mobile phones and other electronic media. These could be used to provide information or behavioural support through websites, CD-ROMs or SMS (text messages).

It is difficult to imagine a country in the Western world without mass media, as it provides a 'constant backdrop' to the societies in which we live (Seale 2002). 'Mass media plays several important functions in society, including providing information, entertainment, articulating and creating meaning, setting agendas for individual and societal discourse and influencing behaviour' (Grilli et al. 2006: 2). As a health practitioner, the use of mass media in relation to health promotion is of particular importance because it remains a medium that is widely used in conjunction with the principles of health promotion. Seale considers that health practitioners are expected to 'deliver accurate, objective information about health risks and health behaviour' (2002: 3) through the media. Alongside this, health practitioners also have a role in *agenda setting* and changing ◀◀ attitudes (Naidoo and Wills 2000) that can be achieved through media use.

Activity 4.1: Media in health promotion

1 List as many recent health promotion mass media campaigns as you can.
2 Of the list that you have identified, what categories do they fit into under the following headings (choose the best-fit category)?

- Promotion of healthy behaviours.
- Risk reduction.
- Health protection.
- Health education.

Tones and Green (2004) consider that there are currently four main areas of debate in health promotion in the use of mass media:

1 Mass media as an unhealthy influence, for example, promoting behaviours that are health damaging (tobacco, alcohol and others).
2 The marketing of unhealthy products, for example fast food.

3 The use of mass media via social marketing.
4 The division between 'selling health' versus 'giving choices'.

The first point includes the role of the mass media at large. Mass media can promote health-damaging behaviours, and thus the goal of health promotion in utilizing media and general mass media use embody contradictory aims. Point 2
can also be included under this umbrella. Mass media as a whole generally does
not print health stories through a concern of the promotion of health and the prevention of ill health, but rather because they are newsworthy, topical, warrant
public attention or attract public interest (Naidoo and Wills 2000).

Points 3 and 4 refer to the design of mass media campaigns using social
marketing. Social marketing raises debates around the use of media, as social
marketing employs principles designed to 'sell' health to populations. The use of
mass media to sell health has been proclaimed to go against the health promotion principles of providing choices and enabling people to make their own decisions, and thus remains an area for contentious debate.

COMMON MASS MEDIA USE IN HEALTH PROMOTION

Television and video

Most mass media relies on large mass media mechanisms such as television or
radio (Atkin 2001), and this is supported by Risi et al. (2004) who indicate that
television is the leading source of media information about health issues.
Television has been found to have some positive effects in health promotion; for
example, in an examination of mass media use among recent quitters of smoking, television advertisements were identified as the most helpful to those trying
to stop smoking (Beiner et al. 2006). Chew et al. (2002) found that a health promotion television series in Poland increased knowledge and enhanced health
beliefs around general family health information. Video programmes have also
been found to be among the most successful strategies to improve communication with patients in general practice, and they show a consistent increase in
short-term knowledge (Leiner et al. 2004).

Radio

Radio has been used to promote health through advertisements, education–
entertainment (or edutainment) programmes, and in public service announcements
(PSAs). The use of edutainment is showing rising popularity in developing
countries in particular, and refers to the use of educational messages integrated
into a fictional context. Farr et al. (2005) describe successful results of the use of
entertainment-education in Ethiopia through a soap-opera style radio drama focussing on modern family planning, including HIV/AIDS and risk avoidance. This is
comparable to a study by Vaughan and Rogers (2000), who examined a similar

programme in Tanzania and found progress in adoption of family planning strategies. Wray et al. (2004) also use a radio serial to prevent domestic violence in an African-American community, although effectiveness was mixed, and further exposure analysis and recall was suggested. In the UK, programmes such as 'The Archers' (a radio soap-opera) have created a number of storylines around health issues such as breast cancer (TeHIP 2005), indicating a move towards the use of entertainment–education principles. One alternative way of using the radio is through PSAs. These are free ways to utilize media and are not as commonly used in the UK as in other countries, such as the US. There has been some reported success of these announcements, for example, Meyer et al. (2003) use PSAs to promote gun safety and found that recall of gun safety practices was higher in those exposed to the messages.

Print-based media

Leaflets are one of the most common ways to use media and have shown some consistent results in raising health awareness. Dyer et al. (2005) found that a nutrition education leaflet improved nutritional knowledge in patients at risk of colorectal symptoms, and Humphris and Field (2004) found that a patient information leaflet reduced anxiety about oral health screening. There is less evidence to support the idea that leaflets can change behaviour. Guilera et al. (2006) found that although a leaflet aimed at women with osteoporosis increased health awareness, it did not increase adherence to therapy. Other print-based media can include comics, cartoons, posters or flyers, although Risi et al. (2004) found that the use of photo-comics did not increase screening uptake in a township in South Africa. Unfortunately these areas are currently under-researched and their effectiveness remains questionable. Another area that has received attention in print media is the use of warning labels on cigarette packets. O'Hegarty et al. (2006) found that warning labels are used to promote interest in quitting, and also propose that text plus graphic warning labels (such as those in Canada) may be more effective than text only (used in places like the UK).

Multi-media

Research suggests that the use of a selection of mass media channels is more likely to result in an effective campaign (Tones and Green 2004; Peterson et al. 2005). Russell et al. (2005) suggests the use of multiple media options to reach the proposed audience. For example, in a student population, flyers, email, induction packs and on-campus stalls may be better than a more traditional solo medium of posters or newspapers. 'Soul City', the ongoing South African education–entertainment campaign utilizing radio dramas, photo-comics, posters, billboards and other media (although on a large scale) is said to have yielded positive results in a variety of health topics (Singhal and Rogers 2001). Usdin et al. (2005), for example, illustrate how 'Soul City' successfully reached groups by television, billboards and printed booklets to prevent gender-based violence. They found an increase in awareness; for example, more people were aware of the telephone help-line, and they also found an attitude shift in domestic violence, where more people thought domestic violence was not a private affair.

McAlister et al. (2000), in their community-based campaign, found a reduction in smoking through a large-scale 'quit and win' competition. The use of traditional mass media methods (for example leaflets) alongside local media (such as success stories about those who have managed to quit) were seen as essential to achieving success. However, it is not always clear that multi-media use results in more success, particularly when the campaign has concluded. Smith et al. (2002) found that during a television and print 'sun safety' campaign there was increased knowledge of some sun safety behaviours and some increase in sun-protection behaviours. This was not sustained after the campaign had concluded, suggesting multi-media may only herald short-term effects. It is also important to remember that the difference between some of the larger multi-media campaigns is their heavy resource base (for example funding, facilities, resources), something small-scale campaigns may not have.

Case Study 4.1   Hedgehogs

The UK Department for Transport (DfT 2006) uses multi-media for one of its road-crossing campaigns for children. The Hedgehogs campaign (see Figure 4.2) is aimed at primary school children to help them gain road-crossing skills. Alongside a variety of print materials (for example posters, songs and leaflets), there is a children's website where children and their hedgehog 'friend' practice road safety. See www. hedgehogs. gov.uk for more information.

Case Study 4.2   Mass media, tobacco use and young people

- Bates et al. (2003) propose that a national tobacco campaign should include public communication programmes which use mass media, and that these should be used to de-normalize and create an emotional response in smokers. They recommend giving a low priority to school-based initiatives, youth access initiatives (restricting access to under-16s, for example), and youth 'counter-marketing' strategies (which can strengthen appeal to cigarettes).
- Farrelly et al. (2003) consider that anti-tobacco advertising campaigns have been demonstrated to have the potential to decrease tobacco use among young people, although these campaigns demonstrate more success when combined with school or community programmes. This finding is fairly consistent for campaigns at a larger level.
- Sowden and Arblaster (2006) conclude that the evidence is not strong for mass media deterring young people from starting smoking.

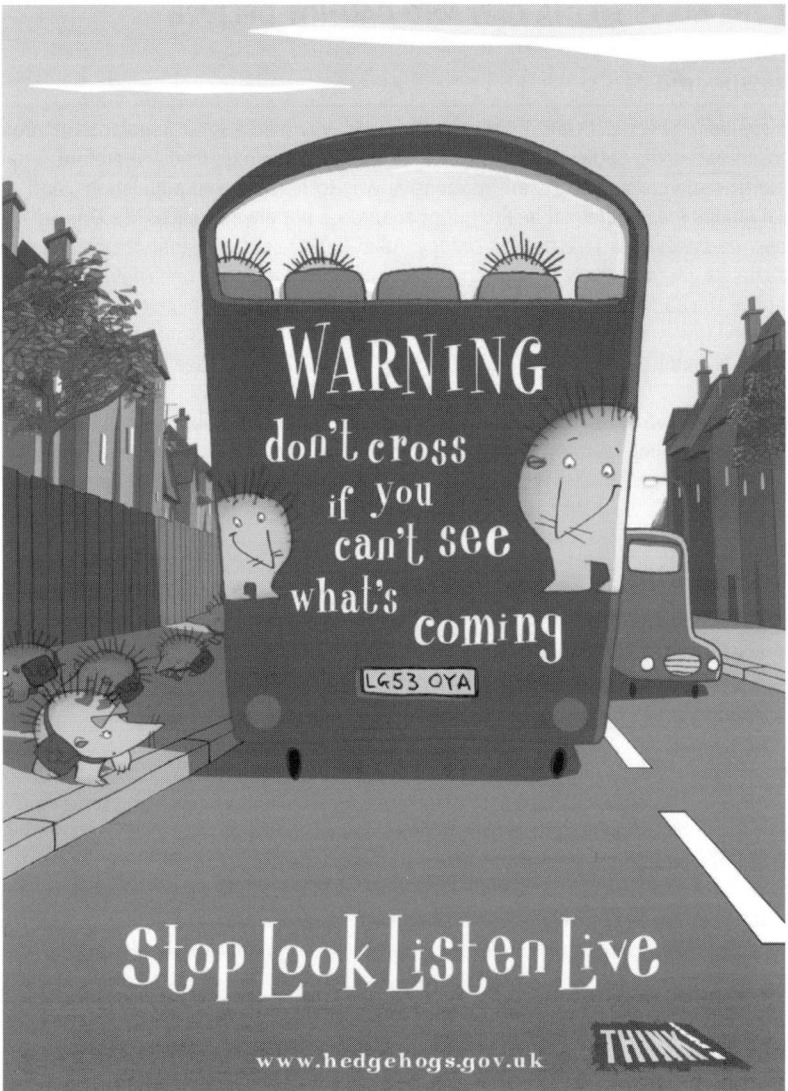

Figure 4.2   The UK Department for Trade and Transport's THINK! Road Safety Hedgehogs Campaign for Children (DFTT 2006a)

Activity 4.2:   Mass media and tobacco

Based on the evidence in Case Study 4.2:

1   How do you think mass media should be used (if at all) to prevent tobacco use in young people?
2   What methods could you combine (or use instead of) mass media?

WHAT THE MASS MEDIA CAN AND CANNOT DELIVER

The mass media can

- *Achieve wide coverage:* One of the main reasons why media is so popular is its promise of exposure to a wider audience. One distinct advantage of the mass media, therefore, is its potential large-scale coverage. It is an inexpensive way to reach whole populations, and can also reach groups that traditional health information does not always reach (MacDonald 1998).
- *Impact on behaviours receptive to change:* Atkin (2001) considers that campaigns which use mass media are more likely to have an impact if they are looking at behaviours that are already receptive to change. This might include maintaining a healthy behaviour that is already being performed (for example, using sun-cream in the sun) or a behaviour that requires little persuasion (for example, eating more fresh fruit and vegetables in a diet already rich in fruit and vegetables).
- *Convey simple information:* Mass media can convey simple information and change behaviour if there are enabling factors (Naidoo and Wills 2000). For example, a message that encourages physical activity five times a week could change the behaviour of someone who currently exercises three times a week who has a subscription to a local gym, who would then have two extra sessions for no extra fee.
- *Increase knowledge:* Mass media can increase knowledge (Naidoo and Wills 2000). Barbor et al. (2003) found that mass media campaigns around alcohol and drugs have been found to increase knowledge, but not to change behaviour. MacDonald promotes mass media as 'generators of health insight' (1998: 110), suggesting the media has a role in promoting interest and providing information about health-related issues.
- *Put health on the public agenda:* Mass media can help raise health interest in the general public; for example, Cooper et al. (2000) describe the development of a television drama series based on the medical drama programme 'ER', providing a forum to discuss health concerns raised in 'ER'. This proved to be a successful arena for highlighting topics that were timely public health issues based on current television programmes. Media advocacy (discussed later in this chapter) and utilizing the media for free via newspapers or magazines can increase public awareness of health issues. Grilli et al. (2006), for example, found that mass media can encourage the use of health services and that both planned and unplanned media coverage can change health service use, suggesting that key decision makers should take an interest in media use.

Case Study 4.3   Breastfeeding. Good for baby. Good for mum

The Health Promotion Agency in Northern Ireland in 2004–5 ran a campaign that aimed to raise public awareness of the health benefits of breastfeeding and to promote breastfeeding as socially acceptable in order to encourage a wider uptake of breastfeeding. Television and radio advertising was used, as well as advertisements on buses and posters. The television strap-line was 'Breastfeeding. Good for baby. Good for mum.' This strap-line intended to focus on the first aim (raising awareness of health benefits). The radio and posters had the strap-line 'Breastfeeding mums need your support – because every baby deserve the best'. This strap-line aimed to cover the second objective: to promote breastfeeding as socially acceptable.

(HPA 2004)

It is still hotly debated just how much the mass media can achieve. Research suggests that there are some areas where mass media is not an appropriate method, as explained below.

The mass media cannot ...

- *Change structural, political or economic factors:* Myhre and Flora (2000) argue that communication via mass media cannot change structural factors, policies or increase services. In relation to issues that effect whole population groups, for example infectious disease, the mass media is powerless to change structural factors or increase services to decrease rates of infectious disease.
- *Change behaviour without facilitating factors:* Mass media finds it difficult to illicit any behaviour changes in individuals if there are no enabling factors (Naidoo and wills 2000) and any claims to the contrary are often 'exaggerated' (MacDonald 1998). The media often ignore important elements such as social and political contexts that restrict choices or behaviour changes (MacDonald 1998). These could include access to services, economic factors or lack of time, resources or skills.
- *Provide face-to-face support:* One of the advantages of mass media is that it reaches a mass audience. This characteristic results in the mass media being unable to provide any one-to-one support to change behaviours (for example stopping smoking) or to facilitate interpersonal contact (Tones and Green 2004). On the positive side, the move to include helpline numbers, SMS (text messaging) services and websites as part of media campaigns can increase the level of individual support.
- *Teach a skill (or skills):* Seale (2002) proposes that mass media is ineffective in teaching skills. The very nature of media (one message to all) mitigates against teaching a skill, and thus other communication methods need to be used to facilitate acquirement of a skill.
- *Convey complex information:* Mass media cannot convey any complex information (Seale 2002; Naidoo and Wills 2000); simple messages are more appropriate for the media. For example, mass media would find it difficult to convey information about risks of Type II diabetes, its diagnosis, risk factors and management to the whole population in one message. On the other hand, simple messages can be very effective (see Case Study 4.5).
- *Change strong attitudes or beliefs:* Mass media cannot challenge strong beliefs (Seale 2002) or 'shift' attitudes and beliefs (Naidoo and Wills 2000). The role of attitudes and beliefs is often deeply ingrained (see Chapter 2), and mass media alone will find it hard to change these.

It has been suggested that to counter-balance these advantages and disadvantages, a number of strategies may be utilized. First, a combination of methods should be employed. Mass media should be used in conjunction with other programmes that contain interpersonal interactions, such as community-based programmes, and should acknowledge environmental and societal limitations (Tones and Green 2004; Naidoo and Wills 2000). MacDonald argues that mass media has 'immense potential as part of the intersectoral apparatus in promoting health and in enhancing both community and individual empowerment' (1998: 111). This suggest that mass media has a key role to play in health, but only when combined with an integrated approach that utilizes other agencies, resources or methods.

Second, the planned campaign needs to have realistic expectations about what it can achieve in line with the programme aims. If a programme wants to teach a skill, for example, physical activity chair exercises for older people, mass media might not be appropriate. However, if a programme wanted to raise awareness of risks of skin cancer through basic sun safety, mass media could be the appropriate choice.

Activity 4.3:   Suitability of methods for mass media

1   Decide which of these activities could be achieved through the mass media.
2   For those that are unsuitable for mass media, which methods would you suggest instead?

a)   Raising awareness of risk factors in CHD in males above 40.
b)   The opening of a national new 'stop smoking' help-line.
c)   Increasing the number of young women who are screened for cervical cancer.
d)   Enabling young children to have the skills to cross the road safely.
e)   Changing negative attitudes to schizophrenia.

CREATING A HEALTH CAMPAIGN USING MASS MEDIA

It has been suggested that there are conditions that can help to facilitate a successful campaign. Randolf and Viswanath (2004) suggest that developing theory-based campaigns that are clearly evaluated (for example, assessment of exposure) should enable achievement of the campaign outcomes. These include creative and supportive environments, use of theory and analysis and evaluation (Randolf and Viswanath 2004). Noar (2006) adds to this list identifying formative research, segmentation of the audience and message targeting as other key variables of a successful campaign.

Recent campaigns increasingly use theory, and hail theory as an essential factor in the success of a campaign. Randolf and Viswanath (2004) propose that theory can be used to identify the main determinants of behaviour, create appropriate messages and help to choose places for the messages themselves. Sowden and Arblaster (2006) additionally suggest that campaigns should be guided by theoretical constructs.

Understanding of the determinants of behaviour targeted in a campaign could lead to the desired health behaviour being performed (Randolf and Viswanath 2004). As behaviour is influenced by factors defined in theories, it is helpful to choose a theory that fits to the aim and objectives of the campaign (see Chapter 1), alongside wider socially, psychologically and culturally appropriate messages (see Chapter 2). Marcus et al. (1998) suggest that social marketing, the trans-theoretical model and social cognitive theory are influential in developing media-based interventions. Chapter 1 gives detailed advice on using theoretical models in health promotion campaigns.

Campaigns utilizing mass media that are targeted at a certain group of the population can have a modest impact, although this varies between the behaviour that is being targeted, the response of the target group to the mass media and the message that is being sent (Atkin 2001). Effectively researched, well-planned and developed campaigns have higher success and are more likely to last longer (Sowden and Arblaster 2006; Farrelly et al. 2003). Noar (2006) proposes that the

1	**Conduct formative research (pre-target group)** Examine evidence base Consider rationale for campaign
2	**Use theory** Framework and foundation to the campaign
3	**Segment audience** Identify target group demographics including social and psychological factors, social marketing strategies
4	**Message design** Aims/objectives of campaign Targeted to segment audience Choose novel, creative methods
5	**Use chosen/appropriate channels from target group** Medium, exposure, duration
6	**Transmit message** Send the message via the correct channels
7	**Conduct evaluation; process, impact and outcome** Check implementation, exposure, recall and effectiveness Match to campaign objectives

**Figure 4.3   Designer success, based on Noar's (2006) principles for
effective design of mass media campaigns**

more a campaign designer adheres to the principles behind an effective campaign design, the more success can be seen in the uses of mass media in health campaigns. There is increasing evidence that media in campaigns can be effective, providing that programmes adhere to the principles of the campaign design (Noar 2006).

Figure 4.3 illustrates the basic campaign design steps that should be included in a mass media campaign. Although this is a simplified version of processes that a health practitioner would undertake, it provides a checklist of key stages in campaign design. First, it is suggested that pre-research is conducted to determine the target group and the rationale for the campaign. Locating existing literature and examination of the evidence base is also important. Second, the use of theory should be employed. The theoretical models as described in Chapter 1 can be adapted and applied to programme design. The third stage is audience segmentation. This includes identifying the target group's *demographics*, influential social and psychological factors, and may also include social marketing principles. The fourth stage is designing the message. This includes formulating the aims and objectives of the campaign, and then designing and testing a message for the target audience. The fifth stage is the selection of appropriate mass media channels, and how the information will be transmitted through these channels including length, duration and timing. After transmission of the message the last stage includes conducting an evaluation to check the implementation of the message, exposure and recall to enable determination of the success of campaign objectives.

All health campaigns should include an evaluation plan. It is difficult to measure effectiveness (Hill 2004) and exposure levels are often estimated, although this does not always give a true measure of what has been achieved. Recall and recognition measures would help the designer to see how successful the message was in achieving exposure (Randolf and Viswanath 2004). See Chapter 7 for more information on evaluating health promotion work.

SUPPORTIVE ENVIRONMENTS

Campaigns that take the wider environment into consideration are more likely to be achieved, and sustainable in the long term. Myhre and Flora (2000) consider that mass media campaigns should also aim to include communities, rather than just focussing on individuals; for example, in HIV campaigns they propose that mass media should increase the importance of prevention, frame HIV as a community issue, improve 'discourse' around HIV and improve the nature of participation in HIV. An effective mass media campaign for HIV therefore would have to collaborate with interventions that are aimed at improving structural, economic or environmental conditions of a community or communities. Other campaigns have taken these ideas onboard and used them in their work. Figure 4.4 provides an example of The Samaritans' campaign, which aimed to improve discourse around mental health, setting mental health in the context of a current popular television programme.

Environment in the widest sense could include aspects such as schooling or education. Mbananga and Becker (2002) suggest that poor cognitive skills can result in non-understanding of messages, and the importance of a formal education as a foundation for individuals and groups is seen as a link to imparting effective information to groups. This suggests that the addition of education into the wider environmental and societal area may be important in interpreting health promotion messages through the media.

Activity 4.4: Supportive environments – environments and economics

1   As a health practitioner, how would you do the following?

   a) Encourage children to take more exercise when there are no safe environments in their locality.

   b) Advocate household hygiene when there is no money for cleaning products.

   c) Encourage screening uptake when a screening service is under-resourced as it is not a government priority.

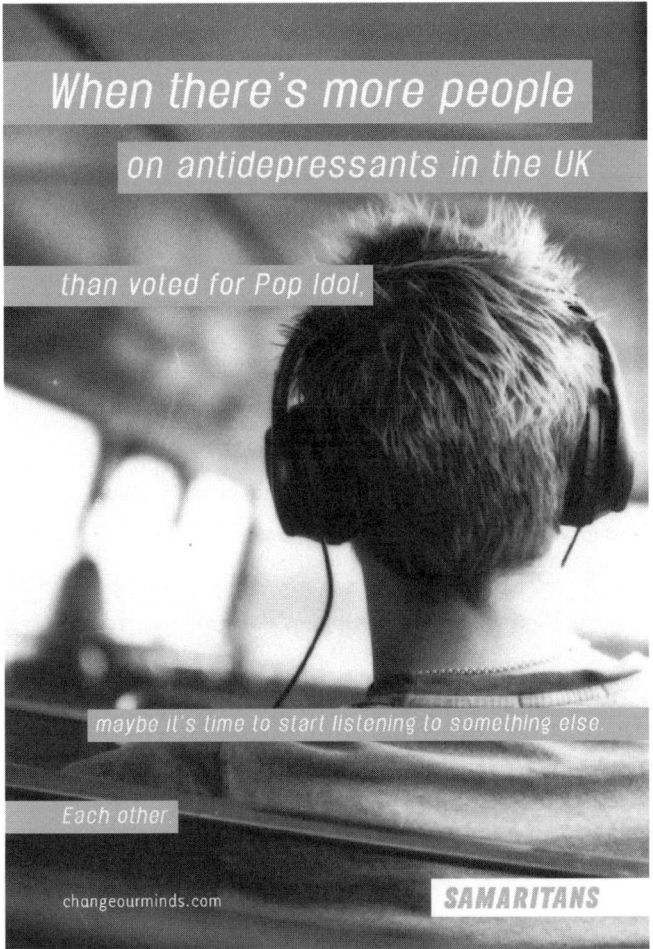

**Figure 4.4   The Samaritans' 2002 'Change our Minds' campaign ©
Samaritans 2006a**

AUDIENCE SEGMENTATION AND MESSAGE DESIGN

Peterson et al. (2005) suggest clear identification of the target group to enable design of phrases that will motivate them: 'for a target group to be aware of a campaign … it must be memorable' (Peterson et al. 2005: 438), therefore choosing and creating an appropriate message is essential. Message pre-testing is vital to counteract any identified negative impacts or unplanned effects of a message. MacDonald (1998) adds that with hard-to-reach groups, pre-testing is paramount. Pre-testing should include checking to see if the message is salient, understood and memorable (Russell et al. 2005), alongside the more traditional message testing of reception, comprehension and response to the message.

1	**Conduct a readability test using members of the target group** Can your target group understand all the words and their meanings? Is the material logical? Consistent? Coherent?
2	**Re-write complex information including unusual or difficult words, and remove any 'jargon'.** Which parts are complicated or need further explanation? Are the main message(s) simple? Would headings help to segment information?
3	**Use 'our'/'we' to maintain a collaborative voice, rather than 'you'** Does the material seek to make people feel included in the text? Are all the materials in the same style and tense?
4	**Simplify complex tables and diagrams** Are the tables/diagrams necessary? Are they easy to understand from a lay perspectives?
5	**Use a glossary of difficult terms** Are there complex words which may need further explanation?
6	**Re-conduct a readability test and pilot on the target group** Do the target audience fully comprehend the revised material?

Figure 4.5   Brief guidelines for re-writing, or designing written material

Case Study 4.5:   Simple messages in current media

I'll be DES – used by The Portman Group (2005) to promote their 'DESignated driver' campaign.

5 a Day – used by the NHS (2006) for the 'five' fruit and vegetables each day campaign.

Talk to Frank – used by the UK government campaign 'Talk to Frank' (DOH 2006b), which provides drugs information to young people.

Know what you're getting into – used by the Metropolitan Police (2006) for their campaign to advise women not to get into unlicensed taxi-cabs (otherwise known as mini-cabs) in London.

The development of a message, themes and appropriate images needs to be done in close conjunction with the target group (Sowden and Arblaster 2006). An example is the work by The Portman Group, who recommend when targeting messages at young women that the focus should be on what excessive drinking could lead to. These include walking home alone, accepting lifts from people they don't know, as well as unsafe sex and how female appearance can be affected with alcohol and over time (DOH 2004). Bates et al. (2003) suggest choosing propositions, for example 'I worry that if I do not stop smoking I will not see my children grow up', or 'I worry that smoking will harm the health of my baby'. For these propositions themes, images and messages can be developed in close conjunction with the target group.

Case Study 4.6:   Thematic words

Peterson et al. (2005) used thematic words to develop messages to promote exercise in 18–30-year-olds. They asked the target group to write down a two to three word phrase that came to mind in the promotion of exercise. Final chosen words included 'fun' and 'my appearance'. Results suggested that the final theme and design should include a range of fun activities shown to promote health, alongside highlighting that physical activity will help you to 'look good' in a 'party setting' focus.

Activity 4.5:   A sensible drinking campaign message

Using the previous case study, try to develop a campaign message for encouraging sensible drinking in 18–25-year-olds:

1   List as many key words that you can think of for 'sensible drinking' and '18–25', along with motivations to 'drink sensibly'.
2   Choose two or three of these words to use as your main campaign theme words.
3   Try to formulate these into a phrase or slogan that your campaign could use.

Once a message has been formulated, exposure to the message needs to be substantial for there to be any effect (Farrelly et al. 2003). Tones and Green (2004) identify repetition of the message as an important component of mass media; spending time developing a message is fruitless if no-one ever sees it.

Activity 4.6:   Message placement

Where would you place your message to encourage sensible drinking (from Activity 5) to enable repeated exposure to the message?

SOCIAL MARKETING

Social marketing applied to health is 'the systematic application of marketing concepts and techniques to achieve specific behaviour goals relevant to improving health and reducing health inequalities' (NSMS 2006: 1). It uses systematic planning for programmes (Tones and Green 2004) and these strengths can be used to help inform the planning, design and development of communication strategies. In recent years it has been integrated into health campaigns more and more as practitioners realize how the uses of models developed in other sectors could translate into health practice. The recently published *Its Our Health* (NSMS 2006), commissioned by the Department of Health, further serves to emphasize the potential of social marketing to health promotion.

Social marketing is more than just mass communication. It takes into account a wide spectrum of influences, including economics, legal measures and policy (Tones and Green 2004). Social marketing frameworks have proved to be particularly adaptable, and marketing principles can be used in a variety of ways in health campaigns. Social marketing has more to offer than just a framework for a campaign but can be fully integrated into interventions with the full spectrum of social marketing aspects. The advantages of social marketing include 'features' applicable to each stage of the campaign design, for example, clear target group identification. Because social marketing follows a clear framework it becomes easier to identify constraints and enabling factors to performing behaviours. There is growing evidence to suggest that social marketing can improve the impact and effectiveness of campaigns (NSMS 2006). Chapter 8 discusses social marketing and evaluation in more detail.

Some health practitioners have taken social marketing concepts fully on board and have integrated social marketing into health promotion campaigns. For example, in the US, the 'Truth' campaign launched in 2000 aimed to 'build a teen-orientated brand to compete health-to-health with tobacco industry brands' (Evans et al. 2002). The Truth campaign wanted to take the notion of a 'brand' that appealed to young people (in the same way that fashion brands target young people), and move away from the adoption of traditional health education health risk messages.

The success of social marketing is based around a variety of 'features'. These include the segmentation of audiences, consumer research, competition, exchange theory, monitoring and the marketing mix (or the four Ps) and interactions between interpersonal media and the mass media (Grier and Bryant 2005).

Audience segmentation

Social marketing borrows commercial marketing techniques (Hill 2004). This includes identifying target groups and their 'consumer orientation', for example, mothers who smoke and have young children. This group is then thoroughly researched and messages are pre-tested on this group. Social marketing splits populations into subgroups based on psychological and social characteristics and behaviours. In health promotion the same process can be applied to practice in the target group.

Activity 4.7:   Audience segmentation

In sexual health interventions there are a variety of groups that could be targeted for sexual health promotion messages. Using an audience segmentation strategy, these groups would be split into sub-groups.

For example: One group that might benefit from a HIV prevention message could be 11–15-year-old secondary school children. They could be divided into male and female, then sexually active and non-sexually active. In the sexually active group they could further be split into contraceptive users and non-contraceptive users and so on.

(Continued)

Using the example of a sexual health message for HIV:

1 Identify the groups that could be targeted for a HIV prevention message.
2 Choose one of these groups and identify what characteristics (for example, male/female) or behaviours (for example, contraceptive/non-contraceptive users) allow 'segmentation' into further sub-groups.

Consumer research

The concept is that what the consumer wants and needs should form the basis of a social marketing strategy. This means researching the targets group's needs, preferences, opinions, beliefs and other areas that impact on behaviour. The move to include evidence-based practice in health promotion is particularly useful for substantiating these findings.

Competition

Social marketing will have thoroughly researched the competition and what product or service they are offering. In health promotion this could include identifying unhealthy behaviours that compete with healthy ones, as well as examining other health messages that are being marketed.

Exchange theory

It is postulated that consumers buying a product will weigh up the pros/cons or benefits/costs. The product bought will more likely be the one with the greatest benefit at the least cost. These costs are not just financial, but can also include time, pleasure, habit, enjoyment and others. In application to health promotion, the benefits of the behaviour need to be highlighted alongside recognition of the costs. For example, stopping smoking could be something that a person enjoys and uses as stress relief (the benefits and costs of smoking) versus advantageous reasons for stopping, including more money or a clearer complexion (the costs of stopping).

Monitoring

Social marketing uses evaluation from the start of the planning process to the end. In health promotion, evaluation is fundamental to check that programmes are achieving their objectives, and all health promotion programmes should include process, impact and outcome evaluation (see Chapter 8).

The four Ps

In addition to audience segmentation, exchange theories and competition, social marketing also borrows a marketing mix known as the four (or five) Ps. These

Ps are **Product, Price, Place, Promotion**, and sometimes a fifth additional variable **Positioning.** They form the central core of any social marketing plan, and their attractiveness lies in their ease of application to health promotion work.

- *Product:* the characteristics of the product (or behaviour), i.e. attractiveness.
- *Price:* the costs, value and importance of performing a behaviour (actual and imagined), including social, economic, psychological costs.
- *Place:* where the product (or behaviour) is available.
- *Promotion:* where the product is sold, including publicity, message design and distribution.
- *Positioning:* framing issues so that the target group remembers them.

This marketing mix could be applied to health behaviour and campaign design.

Activity 4.8:   The four Ps

Following the four Ps framework described above, apply the framework to the following activity:

A health promotion campaign to reduce salt in diet (the Product) in a 60+ female age-group in a small community.

1   Identify what **P**rice, **P**lace, **P**romotion and **P**ositioning you could use to promote reduction in salt.

CRITICISMS OF SOCIAL MARKETING

Although promising for health promotion work, social marketing is not without its critics. The focus of social marketing on individuals rather than the broader determinants of health have come under some criticism (see Grier and Bryant 2005). Accusations of providing simple problems to complex solutions (MacDonald 1998) alongside the suggestion that health promotion should take more of a social and political focus (Hill 2004) surround the use of social marketing. The individual is the main focus in social marketing, meaning economic or social conditions are often ignored (MacDonald 1998). The most common criticism is that social marketing is 'manipulative' as it persuades people to be healthy in the same way that consumers are persuaded to buy products. This borrowing of what Hill (2004) refers to as 'manipulative techniques' has led to questions around ethical issues of social marketing.

In defence of social marketing, however, the 'consumer research' aspect proposes that the consumer (or audience) define their own wants and needs when 'buying' a product. In health, therefore, involving the target group in all the pre-planning processes enables the target group to 'buy' the healthy product that they want.

Despite social marketing's tendency to be expensive, time consuming and inappropriate for small-scale projects (Grier and Bryant 2005), the principles applied in a social marketing framework do reflect the more traditional planning frameworks in health promotion. This suggests a productive move to ally theoretical principles closely with practice, which is a positive step for health practitioners and their health promotion work.

UTILIZING THE MEDIA FOR FREE

Health in the news and newspapers

Research suggests, from the evaluation of one UK news channel and one newspaper, that the most common type of health story is 'health care' (Harrabin et al. 2003), meaning those that are hospital or primary care based. They further found that very little information was seen to focus on preventive health measures, and there was an imbalance of reporting of stories. Taking a crude measure of death rate, they approximated that there was one news story per 8,571 people who died of smoking in comparison to one news story per 0.33 people who died of vCJD (Harrabin et al. 2003). Given that newspapers often reflect public attitudes and interest, this imbalance should be of interest to the health practitioner. If current media interest is not focused towards health promotion, the general population, policy-makers and governments will also rate cure more highly that prevention.

Newspapers may be one way to place health issues into the public's view. There is evidence that some media coverage impacts on behaviour (for example, health scares), policy can take cues from media, and government priorities take cues from the media agenda (Harrabin et al. 2003). As a health practitioner, raising health promotion issues in newspapers may impact on any of these three processes. Health practitioners frequently under-use sources for generating mass media coverage (Atkin 2001). Taking advantage of news stories or features in local newspapers, for example, could be one way of raising the profile of health promotion issues.

Health practitioners should take an active approach to media use in health promotion and strive to develop this, for example, including stories in the media that appeal to audiences from human interest angles. Smaller communities, with less sources of power, will have more opportunities to influence news as the content is usually a reflection of what is happening in that community (Martinson and Hinderman 2005). Health education or health agenda rising in newspapers also has a low resource implication. In the developing world newspapers may be useful in supplementing other activities (Nishtar et al. 2004) for preventive behaviours. A proactive health practitioner could work towards achieving coverage of a news issue with local community groups as part of the health promotion role.

Activity 4.9: Local newspapers

1   Examine any local or national newspaper and list the ways that health practitioners could use the newspapers to promote health topics, for example, writing a letter to the letters page.

Media advocacy

Media advocacy is the 'strategic use of mass media for advancing social or public policy initiatives' (MacDonald 1998: 116). Media advocacy attempts to change and influence programmes, policies or agendas that can be damaging to
▸▸ health. It has been suggested that print media and *health advocacy* play a strong role in the adoption of policies and laws (Ashbridge 2006), probably through drawing attention to a particular issue that encourages a response from the policymaker. Media advocacy may be one way of utilizing media to raise public awareness or influence public policy from a group or community advocated action. The health practitioners that utilize media advocacy are those 'health activists who confront social rather than individual pathogens' (Tones and Green 2004: 253). Media advocacy therefore is practiced by those practitioners who consider that health is influenced by the wider structural factors in society.

There are some organizations and groups in society that promote disease rather than health, or as Freudenberg notes, 'organizational practices or policies that encourage unhealthy behaviours, lifestyles or environments' (2005: 299). These behaviours can include a variety of factors embodied by organizations who seek to exert power, authority or jurisdiction. 'Advertising, public relations, lobbying, campaign contributions and sponsored research' (Freudenberg 2005: 307) are all ways that large organizations can exert power. They can use media to advertise (unhealthy) products alongside more subtle routes of power, for example by giving funding to a charity, lobbying current governmental departments to support their cause or donating money to fund research. All of these actions have the goal of enabling promotion of their products, thus increasing profits and power.

Activity 4.10:   Media advocacy

1   Make a list current national organizations or groups who promote products that could be classed as health damaging.
2   Choose one of these, and say how using media advocacy techniques described above could advocate a change to these health-damaging behaviours.

Challenging these large organizations can be difficult. Action can include advocating change or influencing organizational practices or policies. This might be through legislative action on the part of the health practitioner or through influencing policy such as restricting the use of advertising. It could also be through responding to news or creating new news items around these health-damaging practices.

One example of this is action aimed at corporations by publicly boycotting products or utilizing existing propaganda and changing it for the purposes of health, also referred to as 'civil disobedience' (Tones and Green 2004).

Organizations such as BUGAUP (Billboard Utilizing Graffitists Against Unhealthy Promotions), an Australian-based advocacy movement use tobacco billboards as a centre of change by 'doctoring' advertisements from tobacco companies. The group change the words or meanings of tobacco promotion advertisements to produce 'doctored' advertisements that portray tobacco as health damaging and sometimes as a habit that is just plain ridiculous.

Education, information and mobilization of campaigns are also influential ways of using media to challenge practice. Counter-advertising, advocacy alongside education and information in community groups can encourage action. As a health practitioner, there are a number of angles that can be taken to challenge organizational practices or policies that damage health. Finding the people inside communities, groups or organizations who make a difference is part of media advocacy. Those who are in a position of influence are more likely to be able to make a difference.

Media advocacy has been challenged by some practitioners who argue that there is little evidence to show these companies are damaging the health of others, and that health promotion should look at individual behaviours rather than the wider sphere of health. Others propose it may jeopardize public relations, funding or the neutral role of the health educator (Freudenberg 2005). Given the fundamental definition of health promotion that includes wider determinants of health, media advocacy is perhaps something that will gain more popularity with practitioners. The role played by new developments in society may require responses that differ from the more traditional role of the health educator. Smoke-free workplaces and bars, an emphasis in new government documentation on workplace health and a focus on at-risk behaviours, tobacco or fast foods are all part of corporate behaviours that can harm health, and something that current-day health practitioners may find they are increasingly expected to respond to.

USING INCENTIVES: FEAR APPEALS AND POSITIVE APPEALS

Health promotion has traditionally conducted messages where audiences usually have to stop doing something, particularly things that are 'comfortable habits … and … pleasurable experiences' (Monahan 1995: 81). Usually messages are designed in health to promote fear or present facts in a rational way, which is contradictory to commercial advertising that rarely uses rational fear-provoking messages but adopts a more positive focus (Monahan 1995). While health messages encourage people to stop smoking or drink sensibly, among other things, commercial marketing is doing the opposite. Commercial marketing encourages these opposing behaviours through entertaining and engaging audiences to utilize, purchase a product or undertake a behaviour by making the product as attractive as possible.

Fear appeals

A fear appeal is 'threatening the audience with harmful outcomes from initiating or continuing an unhealthy practice' (Atkin 2001: 61), usually through a message that emphasizes possible physical harm or social consequences of failing to comply with the recommended message (Hale and Dillard 1995). For example, if you drink and drive you may be involved in a serious accident, or if you smoke tobacco you are more likely to die a premature death.

Atkin (2001) considers that well-designed fear appeals can be quite effective in changing behaviours, although they should also show the audience how to change behaviour. Effective fear appeal messages should include a problem-solution framework (Hale and Dillard 1995). This could be emphasizing the threat and the vulnerability of the target audience to that threat and then providing a solution or recommendations to that problem. Green and Witte (2006) propose that fear arousal messages can work if they are combined with self-efficacy skills that could lead to behaviour change. Rarely, however, do mass media interventions allow for the development of self-efficacy skills. It is important to recognize that not all fear appeals work in all circumstances. Fear appeals that audiences find challenging or troubling will often not reach a target audience (Monahan 1995) and messages that confuse or increase fear may be frequently ignored or difficult to recall.

Activity 4.11:   Fear appeals

You are designing a poster campaign for young women to raise awareness of the risks associated with the so-called 'date rape' drug *Rohypnol* from 'spiked' alcoholic drinks.

1   What risks could you highlight associated with this drug for young women?
2   How would you provide a 'solution' to this problem?

Positive appeals

A positive effect message is one that encourages positive feeling, which could in turn influence behaviour or cognitive processes (Monahan 1995). Peterson et al. (2005) recommend the use of positive re-enforcement and the avoidance of negative messages. Positive appeals can be used in a number of ways; they may want to change audience's current perceptions so the audience view the behaviour from a different perception (for example, turning physical activity from being seen as uncomfortable or tiring to being a way to meet new friends, or something that is fun). Positive appeals could also provide evidence of how performing behaviour will have a positive outcome, for example, a case study which shows how someone going through a behaviour change has a successful outcome. Positive messages are also likely to be more effective when positive attitudes already exist (Monahan 1995), and messages can reinforce the positive aspects of performing or changing a behaviour.

CONCLUSION

Fundamentally, in health promotion, health practitioners should no longer be concerned with debates around whether media works or not. Practitioners need to move forward and think about how the elements of media that do work can be used more effectively. Debates still tend to focus on what mass media can and cannot do, when health practitioners need instead to be moving forward and thinking about what aspects of mass media can be used together to promote health more effectively. A combination of techniques (see, for example, MacDonald 1998) suggests combining social marketing and media advocacy may be one solution, alongside a more proactive approach to media use. In a changing age of media and IT, health practitioners should be taking a forward-thinking role towards mass media campaign design.

Furthermore, campaigns should not attempt to re-do what has already been achieved. Randolf and Viswanath (2004) suggest that campaigns should not try to reinvent the wheel as they are 'merely a waste of resources and are doomed to repeat mistakes of the past' (Randolf and Viswanath 2004). Instead practitioners should look at what already works (particularly those programmes that are based on theory) and use this in future work. The mass media arena is crowded with messages all competing for the same audience (Randolf and Viswanath 2004). The health practitioner needs to ensure that health messages are as effective, well-planned and well-designed as the competition that it is up against to truly promote health effectively.

Summary

- This chapter has analysed the role of mass media in health promotion work, with particular attention to what mass media can and cannot achieve.
- The role of theory, supportive environments and message design has been considered, alongside the uses of social marketing in the mass media.
- Alternative means of mass media use has been explored through media advocacy and utilizing the media via newspapers.
- The place of incentives and fear appeals in health promotion programmes has been discussed.

ADDITIONAL READING

For in-depth coverage of a wide range of aspects of health promotion and public health campaigns (although predominately US based): Rice, R E and Atkin, C K (eds) (2001) *Public communication campaigns, 3rd edition.* Sage. London.

Health promotion planning and development issues and strategies are covered in Tones, K and Green, J (2004) *Health promotion: planning and strategies.* Sage. London.

For detailed coverage of a range of mass media issues: Seale, C (2002) *Media and Health.* Sage. London.

5

Information technology in health communication

Nova Corcoran

Learning outcomes:

- Examine the role of IT applications in health promotion practice.
- Explore the application of IT to health promotion interventions.
- Consider ways to overcome the challenges of IT for health promotion practice.

With increasing global development in information technology (IT) alongside the growing need to tackle challenging health issues, new developments in IT are becoming increasingly pertinent to health promotion. The use of IT in health is appealing and increasingly being used in health care as populations are encouraged to utilize modern technology for health information. Health and illness information is widely available to the general public and health professionals alike through the increasing popularity of applications such as the Internet. One of the main objectives is that IT in health should be striving towards is allowing individuals, groups and communities to gain knowledge and information about health issues that can prevent ill health and promote good health. Health practitioners need to be familiar with strategies that utilize IT to empower, encourage and educate the general public in the bid for health protection, health development and health improvement.

THE ROLE OF IT IN HEALTH

IT generally includes all interactive media. Applications such as CD-ROMs, the Internet, touch-screen kiosks, computer games, mobile phones, digital television and other forms of interactive technology fall under this umbrella. IT has recently joined the realms of mass media and in the future is arguably set to usurp traditional media as the new way to send health messages in the Western world. The use of IT in health promotion is a growing field despite some gaps in research. Currently there are a variety of IT applications that have shown promise, and success, in health promotion communication.

The combination of IT applications that work to improve health has sometimes been referred to collectively as *e-health*. E-health includes telecommuni- ◀◀ cation or computer-assisted IT that plays a role in health. These applications have been hailed as offering 'unprecedented opportunities for improving equity in access to heath-enhancing global ... interventions' (Kirigia et al. 2005: 10). This is an optimistic view that suggests a wealth of opportunities for IT. Eysenbach (2001) proposes e-health as an emerging way of thinking rather than a specific list of technologies with an overarching aim to utilize and improve the application of IT. Either definition suggests that e-health is an electronic application with the potential to enhance health. For the purpose of this textbook this definition will exclude aspects that are linked to financial, administrative or clinical data, for example, electronic patient records, telemedicine or decision support systems. IT holds a number of benefits and challenges to both the lay person and the health practitioner and has been framed as offering opportunities to promote health as well as facilitation of access to health and education needs (Fors and Moreno 2002). A clear understanding of what IT is capable of achieving, and what barriers might be in the way of this goal, is necessary for all practitioners with an interest in health.

IT in communication has been used for a variety of health topics to deliver diverse health messages using a range of media. There are a number of domains where health promotion can make use of IT. Fotheringham et al. (2000) suggest two: educating health care practitioners and delivering health behaviour change via the Internet. In addition to these two areas, IT can be used to:

- relay information;
- enable informed decision-making;
- promote healthy behaviours including preventive aspects, for example screening;
- promote support, for example peer information exchanges, emotional support or social support;
- promote self-care, risk reduction or self-help;
- manage demand for health services; and
- facilitate communication.

Activity 5.1:   How could IT be used to ...?

List ways in which you think IT could:

1   Facilitate communication.
2   Promote an information exchange.

One of the distinct advantages of IT is the engagement of the audience. Unlike mass media where the audience is seen as a passive receiver of messages, the very nature of IT requires engagement from the user (see Chapter 4 for in-depth coverage of mass media). This way of accessing information from a health promotion perspective enables the user to be actively engaged in information seeking. IT can provide 'increased learning, information seeking, information processing, and individualised knowledge' (Rice 2001: 28), all processes which form the basic ethos of empowerment in health promotion.

THE PRACTITIONER AND THE LAY PERSON

IT in health promotion promises benefits for both the health practitioner and the lay person.

For the health practitioner

IT holds promise for major changes in the way information is transferred between the health practitioner and the general public (Benigeri and Pluye 2003). Eysenbach (2001) proposes that the move in e-health (and thereby anything remotely connected to IT) includes a list of other 'e's which e-health strives to achieve: efficiency, evidence-based, empowerment, education, extending scope and equity. All of these 'e's are part of the 'e-health' movement and embody the aims of the application of IT to health. As health practitioners work towards goals of enabling, empowering, advocating or mediating health, it is clear to see how IT can help a practitioner in the achievement of these goals that embody the principles of e-health.

For health promotion, the Internet has a use for health professionals as a research and dissemination source (Duffy 2000). This includes research collaboration and dissemination, alongside making it easier to exchange good practice, particularly at local level where research can be difficult to locate through traditional channels.

For the lay person

One of the most hailed advantages of IT over the mass media is the move away from receivers being passive recipients of messages towards becoming an active audience. Mass media traditionally directs predominately a one-way message. Interactive media, however, can involve participation, experimentation, goal development and other audience-centred methods that were previously impossible via mass media (Lieberman 2001). This shift in information seeking in health can be seen as a move towards the fusion of target group involvement in decision-making processes. Users can choose via Interactive IT applications that allow them to be actively supported in a health behaviour change or illness. These can include email, calendars, support groups or disease management (Benigeri and Pluye 2003), all of which include engagement of the target group.

IT has also been quick to utilize its own advantages in the health promotion field. For the lay user, social support networks in the form of chat rooms, email, discussion or question-and-answer pages can be found on most good health promotion websites or CD-ROM packages. The interactive nature of communication in IT allows content to be adapted, altered or tailored to individual users. Provision of information without face-to-face contact is seen as a considerable benefit of IT alongside providing information for hard-to-reach groups (for example, geographically far apart). This allows populations who are geographically far apart to access the same information worldwide.

THE POTENTIAL OF IT IN HEALTH PROMOTION

The desire to use IT in health has arisen due to a variety of challenges rather than one single reason. Wallace (1998) lists several, including the rising costs of health care, changing demographics (for example, an aging population), developments in IT and increasing public pressure to include other forms of health care (for example, complementary medicine). Other challenges may include changing global networks and new health and disease patterns. New technology use is growing in nearly all aspects of health communication (Suggs 2006). Now patients who visit their general practitioner can go armed with more health information (Hall and Visser 2000), and health practitioners are expected to respond accordingly to the newly informed patient.

It is an exciting time for IT in health promotion. 'Technology is no longer the major barrier holding us back from … using IT in health … it is human and organizational issues underlying information management and communication in our health care system that provides the greatest challenge' (Wyatt 1998: 116). Health practitioners are increasingly expected to be engaged with these e-health applications in their daily work. Atkin (2001) argues that the interactive nature of these new technologies can promise a significant advantage over traditional media channels because the message can be tailored or customized to the individual's capabilities, readiness to change stage, style, levels of knowledge and current variables that impact on behaviour such as beliefs. If this is the case, then health promotion needs to make sure IT is used effectively to reap these benefits.

IT for health promotion has utilized a number of media. The most popular in current research and practice is the Internet. Other computer applications that have been used in health communication campaigns include computer-based interventions, mobile computers, touch-screen kiosks, mobile phones, CD-ROMs and more recently SMS (text messaging via mobile phones).

THE INTERNET

The Internet is one of the more widely researched applications of IT in health. Unfortunately the research directed at encouraging healthy behaviours is slow in coming (Cassell et al. 1998), and Duffy et al. (2002) note that there is still an absence of good evidence on delivering health promotion online. Statistics suggest that around 64 per cent of adults in the UK accessed the Internet in 2005, mostly in a home environment (ONS 2006). The Internet has the capacity to reach geographically large areas and different populations in a relatively cost-effective manner (Cassell et al. 1998), and thus can be seen as an ideal medium to send health messages.

Health information is growing in availability on the Internet (Benigerl and Pluye 2003) and as access and usage has grown, health-seeking behaviours on the Internet have also increased (Cline and Haynes 2001). Duffy et al. (2002) propose that the Internet could potentially be used for health improvement to equip people with information that they need. Gainer et al. (2003) support this proposition, and note the Internet is often perceived as a good educational tool and a valuable information source. They also note that seeking information on the Internet has also become routine practice for users and practitioners.

The Internet, although often grouped with mass media or mass communication, does have characteristics that are shared with interpersonal communication and therefore is a 'hybrid' of mass media and interpersonal communication (Cassell et al. 1998). The Internet can provide 'immediate transactional feedback' (Cassell et al. 1998: 72), alongside having the potential to cover large-scale health promotion interventions, making it advantageous over more traditional forms of mass media.

The World Wide Web and other Internet-based resources share a number of positive characteristics in the field of persuasive communication. Interpersonal interactions are essential for encouraging people to perform healthy behaviours (Cassell et al. 1998). The Internet is something that offers the chance of inter-personal contact. Message boards, for example, can give advice and encouragement and can be important for understanding health-seeking behaviours (Macias et al. 2005). Topics on message boards can be wide-ranging, and given that location is not problematic, different people worldwide can congregate online to discuss the same anxieties, share information or support one another through health changes, illness or health behaviours.

The Internet also boasts widespread access and interactivity (Cline and Hayes 2001) as well as having the benefits of being able to be accessed informally or anonymously (Berger et al. 2005). All these aspects could contribute to an increase in the facilitation of healthy behaviours from searching for information to interacting with others about health issues to improving health. Due to its anonymous environment, the Internet may also encourage health-seeking behaviour for sensitive subjects such as sexual health issues or other issues an individual may find difficult to seek help for; Berger et al. (2005) found that people with stigmatized illnesses are more likely to access the Internet for health information than those without stigmatized illnesses, in particular for psychiatric illnesses. Other potential uses of the Internet could be around sensitive subjects; Gainer et al. (2003), for example, found that usage of their website for emergency contraception was predominately accessed by users of emergency contraception, an issue that may raise sensitivity or confidentiality issues.

Other advantages of using the Internet also include the range of interactive elements (Suggs 2006). The use of message boards, quizzes, games, calculators (for example, alcohol units or body mass index (BMI)) can quickly give a response to the user. Other interactive resources allow a virtual or actual two-way interaction, for example, via web cameras. Users can become involved in their own health choices or illness management and interactivity may also allow users to question their own attitudes, behaviours or beliefs around health issues.

Activity 5.2:   Interactive websites

1 What websites can you think of that use interactive resources to promote health?
2 What sort of resources do they use?

COMPUTER-BASED INTERVENTIONS

Computer-based interventions can include a variety of modes of communication including mobile computers, touch-screen kiosks and information supplied in compact disk forms, for example CD-ROMs. The potential for interactivity is high in each of these areas, and quite lengthy interventions with supporting material can be incorporated and re-visited at any time. Computer-based behaviour change interventions using CD-ROM packages have shown promise in short-term behaviour change (Bull et al. 2001), and computer packages can also help in improving and managing care of existing illnesses (Street and Piziak 2001). According to Burns et al. (2006), computer-based programmes that combine health education with online peer support, decision support or support behaviour change may help meet the needs of people with chronic disease.

Computer-based interventions have the advantage of being able to include activities such as games, simulations, diary keeping, information finding or goal setting. McDaniel et al. (2005) used an interactive smoking cessation intervention delivered in a clinical setting for inner city women. They found participants reported formulating more behaviour-orientated stop-smoking strategies, suggesting the use of interactivity in goal setting. Burns et al. (2006) suggest that interactive health communication applications have been found to improve knowledge, social support, health behaviours and clinical outcomes. There is also some evidence to suggest the improvement of self-efficacy. In part, some of these outcomes have been linked to the interactive components in these programmes, the mix of visual aids, and the opportunity for revisiting information alongside 24-hour access.

Street and Piziak (2001) suggest that for computer applications to be successful they need to be based on theoretical frameworks that take into account all factors that can impact on a programme design, from implementation to evaluation. It is not enough to rely on the software and its mobility or interactive elements to promote health; they should be built into interventions in the same way as other more traditional methods would be and subject to the same rigorous testing.

COMPUTER-BASED TOUCH-SCREEN KIOSKS

Touch-screen kiosks have the advantage of either being taken into a person's home or located in a public space such as a shopping centre, GP surgery, pharmacy or library. Their mobility is convenient for health promotion work or information giving. They have the ability to reach different segments of the population, alongside being available for the user when an individual wishes to access the resource. One of the most common touch-screen kiosks in the UK are the NHS Direct kiosks.

Case Study 5.1   NHS Direct kiosks

NHS Direct kiosks are available throughout locations in the UK as part of the government's NHS Plan (DOH 2000). They can be found in health-related locations such as Accident and Emergency Departments, NHS walk-in centres and pharmacies, as well as non-health locations such as supermarkets and libraries. The kiosks are designed to provide out of hours health support working in conjunction with other NHS services (for example the NHS Direct helpline). NHS Direct kiosks aim to provide the general public with information about NHS services, combined with information about how to look after aspects of health. The information comes from a CD-ROM rather than a 'live' source like the Internet.

Research into touch-screen use has been fragmented. Nicholas et al. (2004) measured the use of a touch-screen kiosk in a general practice, and they found that is was most likely to be used by women, who had more regular visits to the GP in the last 12 months. Harari et al. (1997) found with a touch-screen situated in a community pharmacy that just over one-third of users had not used a computer before, and around the same number who used the touch-screen were over 60 years of age, indicating that older age groups and lack of computer skills may not be a barrier to touch-screen use. In relation to health information, Boudioni (2003) suggests that kiosks can increase accessibility of health information. However, Graham et al. (2002) found no benefit between a touch-screen and the traditional method of leaflets in improving understanding of pre-natal tests among pregnant women, although touch-screens showed some reduction in anxiety about pre-natal testing. Further research would need to be done in this area before any definite conclusions are drawn.

Despite the advantages that the variety of locations can provide, for example access to information for those who may not have access to a computer or are seeking information on a sensitive topic, it has been suggested that location can also act as a barrier. Access to health information in public places may restrict the benefits of convenience, flexibility and access to information of a confidential nature (Fotheringham et al. 2000).

Activity 5.3:   Touch-screen kiosks

A touch-screen kiosk is situated in a rural GP practice. In a survey the practice is finding that high numbers of visitors to the GP practice did not use the kiosk. The kiosk is situated in close proximity to other sources of information in a public place. Most users started using the kiosk without a prompt from staff. Those who felt most comfortable with IT were the most likely to use it.

1   Why do you think visitors to the practice are not making use of the kiosk?
2   What would you do to try to encourage visitors to use the kiosk?

COMPUTER-BASED CD-ROMS

CD-ROMs are a useful computer-based resource that does not require an Internet connection and can therefore be used in any location where access to a compatible computer is available. They can also be used for campaign planning (Rice 2001) or other planning processes that require a logical or sequential framework. Health promotion has utilized CD-ROMs in a variety of ways, but their main disadvantage is that their content needs updating to stay accurate (Suggs 2006), which can be a costly and difficult process.

Case Study 5.2   *Walksmart* CD-ROM

Glang et al. (2005) created an interactive *Walksmart* CD-ROM to increase children's ability to use critical street crossing skills. They used a simulated traffic situation via animation and other interaction methods, which mark a move away from traditional pedestrian safety methods that rely heavily on education. They found that children increased their critical street crossing skills at follow-up. The advantages of the CD-ROM included the elements of reality and engagement with the audience. It was also considered a cost-effective way to allow children to practice street-crossing skills in a safe environment.

MOBILE PHONES

Mobile phones are a new global phenomenon and in Western countries mobile phone use can be as much as 80 per cent (MORI 2005). In the UK there are high levels of mobile phone use in most social groups, although older age groups are less likely to use short messaging services (SMS) (Atun and Sittampalam 2006). Wireless phones outnumber land-lines in some developing countries (Eng 2004) and poor or corrupt management can mean land line costs or services can be expensive. In some countries (for example, Africa) mobile phones can be easier to obtain (Kirigia et al. 2005). Mobile phones have the advantage of voice communication alongside SMS, and increasingly access to email, camera facilities and Internet connections are also available.

Telephone support has been used in interventions as a viable way to support pregnant women who want to stop smoking during pregnancy via peer support (Solomon and Flynn 2005). They also note minimal costs for this intervention. However, given that telephones require a person to be nearby when it rings, and confidentiality is not assured, a newer way of sending health promotion information or support is through SMS applications. Atun and Sittampalam (2006) herald SMS as having the advantage of being able to be used in different languages, messages can be tailored, stored until read, can be an immediate response and responses can be sent anonymously.

Figure 5.1 is an example of The Samaritans' (2006b) campaign that uses a 24:7 (24 hours, 7 days a week) mobile phone texting service. The charity also uses email as a way of supporting anyone who needs emotional support. They first identified the potential for their text-messaging service in their report that found 94 per cent of 18–24-year-olds use mobile phones to send personal messages (Samaritans 2006b), thus providing a rationale for mobile phone support to reach this group.

Recent research has examined the role of SMS applications and health. Atun and Sittampalam (2006) indicate three main advantages: efficiency gains in delivery of health care, benefits to the patient and benefits to public health.

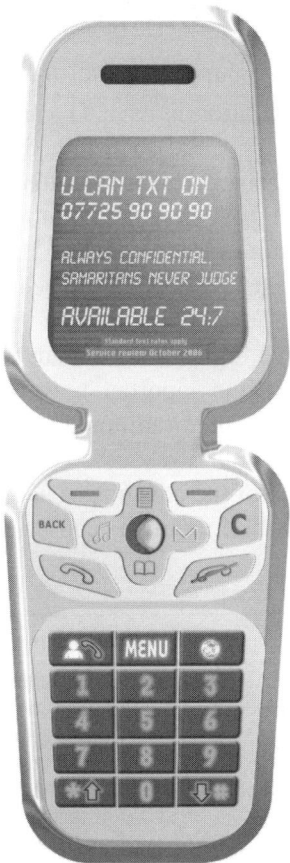

Figure 5.1   The Samaritans' 2006 'txt Samaritans 4 emotional support' campaign © Samaritans 2006a

Efficiency gains can include sending appointment reminders to reduce non-attendance at appointments. It can benefit patient's compliance to medication or treatment routines, such as oral contraceptive reminders. It has been shown to be effective in increasing TB treatment adherence (Atun et al. 2006). The public health benefits of SMS include communicating health information to the public in emergencies, or the ability to send health promotion advice or support.

Activity 5.4:   SMS messaging services

1   What topics do you think might benefit from the sending of SMS messages?
2   What topics do you think are not as suited to sending SMS?

ADVANTAGES AND DISADVANTAGES OF IT

In the emerging field of IT in health communication one of the major factors that should be taken into consideration is what IT can and cannot do. IT, although fast-growing and hailed as essential to health, is not a universal panacea to changing health issues or problems. It is therefore important to consider when communicating health through IT how the communication should be designed, and what the communication is designed for. Health practitioners must take these factors on board and consider how IT can be used to complement or deliver an intervention.

A number of authors have highlighted the advantages and disadvantages of using IT in health promotion. It is important to weigh up the advantages and disadvantages in the same way as other traditional methods. Barriers should be considered before utilizing any online resource or application (Bull et al. 2001). Figure 5.2 summarizes some of the advantages and disadvantage of IT from the findings of Buller et al. (2001), Liberman (2001) and Cassell et al. (1998).

Advantages	Disadvantages
• Time saving • Allows tailoring of information to individual needs • Participatory and interative • Gives choice to targeted person • Allows feedback to targeted person • Can utilize a variety of different mediums (i.e. film, audio, pictures) • Allows application of theoretical models into practice • Economic • Can be user friendly (i.e. touch screen/voice activation)	• No motivation of targeted person to use programmes • Digital divide (i.e. no access to programmes or low literacy) • Competing with other media forms and large companies • Can be costly • Confidentiality and ethical issues need to be addressed

Figure 5.2   The advantages and disadvantages of IT use in health promotion

Overview of advantages

The previous pages have discussed in some detail Internet application advantages, computer-based applications and mobile phones, including the integration of theory and the interactive nature of IT. In addition to these findings, health interventions that utilize online resources or applications have the potential to teach a number of people who would not usually be targeted or may not usually seek health information through the traditional channels (Bull et al. 2001). Seeking IT based health information can be empowering; there are opportunities for building social networks, emotional support and sharing experience through the use of the Internet (Korp 2006). A study by McCoy et al. (2005) proposes that the Internet has potential for self-management education and to promote long-term behavioural change for physical activity and diet, which if true may have potential for the reduction of other lifestyle-related diseases.

Overview of disadvantages

The digital divide refers to the fact that 'well educated and well off have access to and use the Internet to a much greater extent than those who are less well educated and who are less well off' (Korp 2006: 82). Income and education both feature strongly within the notion of the 'digital divide'. The digital divide is not just a country divide, or developed versus developing countries, as this divide can exist within countries. In the UK, for example, around 79 per cent of the highest social classes use the Internet in any location compared to 34 per cent in the lowest social classes (MORI 2005).

According to Korp (2006), the Internet may also promote anxiety in some aspects of health, alongside fostering a narrow definition of health. By focussing on individual aspects of a person's health, the Internet is not encouraging inclusion of wider societal influences. The Internet also promotes vested interest (for example, pharmaceutical companies) of groups who re-enforce the medicalization of health with an emphasis on profits rather than the wellbeing of the individual.

A health practitioner has goals which include giving education around health issues, enhancing health behaviour or empowering individuals, all of which may be contradictory to health websites. Cline and Haynes (2001) draw attention to the creation of health websites for a number of purposes, many of which do not share the same objectives of health promotion. Websites can be created for profit or designed for commercial purposes, promote unhealthy behaviours or contain inaccurate information.

Diversity is an important concept for health promotion practice that should not be neglected in the enthusiasm for working with new forms of IT in health. 'Language proficiency, race, culture and other socio-cultural differences may not be acknowledged' (Cashen et al. 2004: 210) and may make health promotion through IT inappropriate or ineffective when working with diverse groups. Cashen et al. (2004), for example, note that patients with low literacy are less likely to use the Internet and other e-health applications, and traditional broadcast media is still an important information source for some groups and especially those with lower education levels. Information should be made more accessible for those who have the greatest need for information, not just the majority. This may mean designing information for low-literacy levels, in different languages and in different formats in order to reach diverse groups. (Chapter 3 has more information about working with hard-to-reach groups.)

Activity 5.5:   Designing a website

You are working for an organization that targets homeless groups and you want to
design a website that encourages healthy behaviours and practices within homeless
groups who, by the nature of the group, have limited resources.

1   What sort of topics might you want to cover?
2   What sort of language will you use?
3   How would you enable access to the website for this group?

USING IT IN HEALTH PROMOTION

Not all IT applications require the health practitioner to be an experienced IT
user. As a health practitioner, designing resources is an essential part of IT use.
The next section will cover tailoring health promotion materials through IT and
designing resources through a series of design steps. The following section will
also consider alternative ways to involve IT in health promotion. The health
promotion remit extends wider than developing resources; it has a role in
challenging barriers to using IT and addressing issues such as accessibility and
confidentiality to enable users to become involved within IT. The health practitioner may also have a role in encouraging appropriate use of e-health applications. Internet advocacy (as opposed to media advocacy) may be a newer way to
achieving the wider societal goals of health promotion practice.

TAILORING INFORMATION

One advantage of using IT is the potential to include a 'tailored' element, which
is more difficult with traditional forms of media. Tailored information is information that is adapted for individuals and is usually matched to characteristics.
This might be social factors such as demographics and/or psychological factors
such as beliefs or attitudes (see also Chapter 2). The use of tailored information
is supported by the UK government document *Choosing health: making healthy
choices easier* (DOH 2004). This document recommends 'personalization'
or tailoring of health information. In IT messages can be tailored to individuals
rather than a general population more easily than using traditional media
(Suggs 2006). There is room for integration of theoretical constructs into messages, and this can mean that information is more relevant to an individual
person or group of people. The Health Development Agency (HDA 2004) suggest
that targeted and tailored information demonstrates evidence of success in interventions while re-enforcing the suggestion in Chapter 2 that information can be
matched to a clearly identified target group. Current research would suggest that

tailored information does show some benefits over non-tailored information. Oemena et al. (2001) suggest that computer-tailored nutrition education is more effective for motivating change than general education, advocating the use of new technology to deliver tailored messages. Stretcher et al. (2005) also highlight the strengths of web-based tailored support materials in conjunction with nicotine replacement therapy (NRT) over a non-tailored cessation programme. Information around tailoring has been contradictory, for example, De Nooijer et al. (2002) found that for early detection of cancer both tailored and non-tailored information was read by the majority of the groups. They also draw attention to tailored information not being as effective if it is not well matched to characteristics.

Case Study 5.3   Tailoring messages to theoretical models

The transtheoretical model (or stages of change model) has been used in tailoring information to a number of health behaviours. The five stages of change that were specified in Chapter 1 are: pre-contemplation (not interested in change), contemplation (thinking about change), preparation (preparing to change), action (performing the change) and maintenance (maintaining the change).

An example of how the model has been used to tailor messages to those at different phases of change can be illustrated as follows. In smoking prevention the information might be tailored to each stage: those in the contemplation phase might be given a message that says: 'Do you know there is a range of help available to you to help you quit?' Or those in the action stage might be given a message that says 'Well done – you are doing really well at being smoke-free.'

Activity 5.6:   Tailoring messages

You are designing part of a website for encouraging physical activity, based on the transtheoretical model.

1   What messages would you tailor to individuals who are at each of the five phases of the transtheoretical model?

DESIGNING RESOURCES IN IT

If health practitioners want to design IT resources in their health communication strategies, a number of key aspects need to be considered beforehand. These include using the target group in the design and development and integrating theory and evidence into practice. Given that IT (particularly the Internet) is competitive and increasingly commercialized, health promotion needs to make sure the information produced has strong design features and is of a high enough quality (Cassell et al. 1998) to compete in an increasingly growing global health marketplace.

Using the target group

In line with Chapter 2, research indicates that incorporating user beliefs into content delivery together with usability testing is vital (McDaniel et al. 2005). The Internet has traditionally been associated with younger users as the presumption is that they are more IT-literate than older adults. McCoy et al. (2005) found that participants in their 40s and above thought the online delivery of a diet and physical activity programme was not less attractive to older individuals and did not represent a major barrier to participation, thus contradicting previous assumptions. Some studies have also shown that the Internet is a useful tool for reaching the non-traditional users of IT. These examples serve to illustrate that health promotion cannot operate on assumptions, but must involve the target group in the design, development and testing of the resources.

Integrating theory and the evidence base

As outlined in Chapter 1, health education programmes should integrate concepts from theory into the use of IT (Fotheringham et al. 2000). The Health Development Agency (HDA 2004) also suggests the use of theoretical models when developing interventions. CD-ROMs, computer packages or the Internet can assist in the design of programmes that include some of the more popular health promotion theories. Cassell et al. (1998) utilized the health belief model and the transtheoretical model in IT via the Internet, but equally these theories can be applied to other IT media (see Chapter 1 for more detail of these theories). The use of the health belief model could include tailoring messages to benefits and barriers identified by the user or activities around perceived susceptibility and perceived severity (see Activity 5.7). The use of the transtheoretical model could be employed to target different message at different stages of change (see Case Study 5.3).

Activity 5.7:   Health belief model barriers on a website

The health belief model proposes benefits and barriers that are important to health. You are working on a 'look after your heart' website that aims to remove some of the barriers to eating food groups low in fat.

1   List all the barriers you can think of that stop people eating foods that are low in fat.
2   What kind of messages could you give users to try to remove some of these barriers?

Design steps

Lieberman (2001) makes nine recommendations for designing interactive campaigns with young people and adolescents. These include use of appropriate media, use of appealing characters, incorporating challenges and goals, creating functional learning environments, facilitating social interactions, allowing anonymity and involving the target group in design and testing.

---

1 **Include the use of an appropriate media for that target group**
   For example, older adults may not want to play game-based activities, but may be more interested in using discussion boards.
2 **Use role models or creditable sources**
   This could be someone who has performed the behaviour or someone who the proposed target groups can relate to.
3 **Incorporate ways of goal setting**
   Allow space for people to set goals or targets for behaviour change, supporting these goals as much as the software will allow.
4 **Create an environment which is suitable for the topic both in terms of medium used and the style**
   If you are wanting to influence beliefs, a discussions board or real life stories might be helpful; if you are looking to influence attitudes, some interactive feedback mechanisms might be helpful.
5 **Facilitate social interaction**
   Create areas where there is interaction. This could be discussion boards, user stories or ask-a-question areas. Setting up information or forming support networks may help facilitate and support change.
6 **Protecting anonymity and confidentiality**
   It is essential that mechanisms are in place to allow users to make up their own pseudonyms or to receive email feedback but retain confidentiality.
7 **Involve the target group in the design and testing**
   If the target group is involved in the design and testing of the resources and applications, it is more likely to be user-friendly to that group and be used in their intended way.

Figure 5.3 *Seven-step checklist for IT-based resources*

Although Lieberman (2001) applied these stages to young people and adolescents, many of these nine phases could be adapted to suit a more general population for interactive campaigns. Young people and adolescent behaviour may be different than adults' in the emphasis on role models and creating of learning environments when adults may already have these skills. However, learning new skills, influencing attitudes or challenging beliefs are important to adopting new behaviours. *Communicating Health: Strategies for Health Promotion* proposes a similar seven-step formula for general design of IT-based resources (see Figure 5.3). Using appropriate media, role models or credible sources, incorporating goal settings, creating a suitable environment, facilitating social interaction, protecting anonymity and involving the target group should all be included in website design. This seven-step framework helps to overcome some of the barriers associated with IT earlier (for example, confidentiality), and makes use of current research to inform design. Although a specialist IT team will be needed in the set-up and maintenance of the website, health practitioners have a role to play in this team by helping to inform the design and content of websites.

Activity 5.8:   The seven-step checklist for a website design

You are setting up a website on the Internet aimed at promoting positive body image and increasing self-esteem in women from 25 upwards that will be run by your local health promotion department.

  Following the seven-step formula (Figure 5.3), try to answer the following questions:

1   What media sources would you use?
2   What role models or creditable sources might you use?
3   What sort of goal-setting activities might you include?
4   What sort of style would your website adopt (in terms of content, visually etc.)?
5   How would you facilitate social interaction?
6   How might you protect anonymity of users?
7   Where might you go to get a small sample of your target group to become involved in the design and testing?

OVERCOMING BARRIERS TO IT

There is a wealth of health information that utilizes the Internet, CD-ROMs or other computer packages. The role of the health promoter might actually not be the design of new resources or tailored information to individuals, but the removal of barriers that prevent people accessing information in the first place.

Raising awareness

Not all barriers to health information are practical. Bull et al. (2001) suggest that the biggest barrier to STI/HIV information is that people do not think they need such information. In addition to this, McCoy et al. (2005) found that participation in a diet and physical activity programme was discontinued due to behavioural un-readiness rather than technology related reasons. Therefore health practitioners might not be working directly in IT, but will continue to raise awareness of health promotion issues by encouraging access to appropriate information and support.

Accessibility

Korp (2006) suggest that for health information to be truly health promoting, individuals', abilities to evaluate information sources for their own needs and interests could be strengthened. This draws on a different health promotion aim, that of empowering and enabling the individual to be able to find the information they need and evaluate this information for its key properties. Benigeri and Pluye (2003) highlight the need for supported access in homes and public places, and call for a simplification of Internet processes, clear organization of material and a move to integrate health professionals in the processes of interactive communication. Boudioni (2003) suggests that NHS touch-screen kiosks in supermarkets, leisure centres and NHS walk-in centres are used the most as there is a higher proportion of people visiting these locations, thus advocacy for more accessible locations for information retrieval could be part of the health promotion role.

Another barrier to health promotion use of IT is the lack of IT skills in some users. Practical barriers may be important for some groups, and different media of IT may need to be considered. For example, access to IT by a person or groups with disabilities or functional decline may be facilitated by using touch-screens instead of a mouse (Cashen et al. 2004). Other issues could include adequate disabled access to information, alongside visual clarity (for example, information available in a large font).

Activity 5.9: Practical barriers

1   What other practical barriers can you see to accessing information?
2   How might you overcome these?

Empowering practitioners and users

Cline and Haynes (2001) consider that the challenge of IT is to facilitate use of the Internet together with the health care providers, and bearing this in mind to build up an evidence base that supports best use of the Internet. This would suggest that the health practitioner becomes someone who provides information around IT (for example, recommending a CD-ROM or website). Alongside this, health practitioners contribute to the development of an evidence base of best practice. This could take a number of forms, although as Rodrigues (2000) highlights, designing an evidence-based system in health management, service delivery and other health care delivery areas requires time, resources and financial assistance, which remains a major challenge for health practitioners.

Confidentiality

Concerns over confidentiality may be addressed through the design and promotion of applications that have a strong confidentiality policy or regulations in place (Bull et al. 2001). Constant reassurance about Internet security is also important (Duffy et al. 2002). As one of the advantages of IT is confidentiality, it is important to make sure applications ensure anonymity. For example, consider removing anything that asks for personal details and allow users to discuss anonymously or by using pseudonyms.

Quality assurance

Given the concerns over quality of information on the Internet, health practitioners who design information should make sure it is subjected to the same standards as traditional information, which includes quality, trustworthiness and message characteristics (Cline and Haynes 2001). Duffy et al. (2002) propose that information should be reliable, up to date, clear and comprehensive. A study by Hong (2006) suggests that credibility such as expertise and trust were linked to intentions to re-visit websites. This means that information needs to be well managed and constantly checked for accuracy or errors. Provision of a list of your organization's recommended websites would be good practice, along with careful maintenance of ones' own organization's website.

Activity 5.10:   Recommending websites

Think about health websites that you have looked at in your work or study.

1   Which ones would you recommend as good health promotion websites, and why?

INTERNET ADVOCACY

The Internet contains a wealth of information, and given that freedom is something that embodies the ideology of the Internet, there will be information available that can both promote and damage health. Multinational companies, organizations, groups and individuals can use the Internet and therefore any topic of their choice can be covered. A proportion of these topics can encourage, promote or facilitate behaviours that could impact on individuals or groups in a negative way. Promotion of cigarettes, pharmaceutical drugs, alcohol use or illegal substance use, for example, are products that can be marketed at the Internet user but may in turn have a negative health impact. Tobacco and alcohol promotion can glamorize smoking or alcohol and target younger age groups, and in some countries provide access to these products. It is also a mistake to assume that promotion of unhealthy products is from the companies and promoters only. There are clubs, chat-rooms, web pages and websites dedicated to cigarettes, alcohol and illegal substance use run by (and for) those who participate in these lifestyle choices.

Internet advocacy is one way a health practitioner can challenge the promotion of healthy products. Similar to media advocacy in principle (see Chapter 4), the Internet can be used as a source of campaigning for change (Ribisl 2003). Environmental pressure groups have already taken up this idea, and you can now send an electronically generated letter to a local MP or a corporate group to pressurize them into changing unhealthy policies or practices. Another way of utilizing Internet networks is by use of e-cards or e-postcards, which encourage people to send a message on to others.

The role of the health practitioner must be to compete alongside these messages to make sure that healthy messages also reach populations. Something that is under-used but is seeing more and more media attention in a non-health setting is the use of Internet blogs (diary-style-Internet based information) or the creation of clubs, which currently are used by the online community. Ribisl (2003) draws attention to the use of teenage smoking clubs online. The use of Internet blogs and the creating of clubs in health promotion issues are yet to be explored fully. Given that they exist in health-damaging behaviours, the creation of counter-clubs for young people may be a possibility, and Internet blogs of those who are going through a health behaviour change may be a counter-response.

Other means of Internet advocacy may be encouraging the use of filters, blocking or regulating technology (i.e. parental control mechanisms) as well as the more difficult task of monitoring health-damaging behaviours.

CONCLUSION

Eng (2004) proposes that the future of IT includes newer ways to increase disease surveillance and control, environmental and pollution monitoring, food safety, self-care and population screening. IT has the potential to become part of the global changes in health. In countries that still have restricted or limited access to IT, the role of IT to promote health can only remain limited. In some developing countries there is a need for high-impact interventions, although currently technology in developing countries is fragmented, or lacks clear infrastructures (Eng 2004). Until this digital divide is addressed, there cannot be fair access to health for all. IT must co-exist along with more traditional means of delivery and a sense of realism needs to be maintained in order to include those who are unable to access the IT revolution.

There is now a presumption that interactive and multi-media health communication is better or more superior than traditional means of health communication (Street and Piziak 2001). Research into IT is still on-going, and given the array of contradictory or under-researched areas, it will be several years before research is conclusive. By far the best way for a practitioner to proceed is to investigate target groups' preference; this way communication is more likely to reach those for whom it is designed. It must be remembered that it is not necessarily suitable for all interventions or for all target groups.

Burns et al. (2006) suggest the role of emotional, clinical or economic outcomes have been under-researched. This also applies to research in newer areas, for example, SMS and health or the use of Internet applications. Currently being trialled in the US are 'Health Risk Appraisal (HRA) packages'. These are patient filled-in and are an adaptation of a health risk questionnaire. The software utilizes decision support software and can produce personalized health information to users. Iliffe et al. (2005) propose that this may have the benefit of reducing time costs for practitioners, and allows for tailoring of health promotion information to different *at-risk groups*.

Other under-researched areas include the new ways that IT has been revolutionising health care. 'Telemedicine', a general term that refers to a wide range of technologies and applications (Demiris et al. 2005) that allows medical information to be exchanged between different places and enables treatment to be provided at a distance, may have future impacts on health promotion. These include cost of care, quality of care and access to care (Demiris et al. 2005). The role of this mechanism in health promotion and health education remains to a large extent unknown. Other applications could include clinical information systems, such as clinical decision support systems, electronic patient records or smart cards (a card that contains patient information), which will all have a role to play in the wider spectrum of health promotion and public health. We are in a global age of changing technology where anything could happen, and practitioners will need to stay ahead of developments in order to truly promote health effectively.

Summary

- This chapter has considered the advantages and disadvantages for using IT in health.
- It has considered the role of the Internet, mobile phones and computer-based technology (CD-ROMs and touch-screen kiosks).
- This chapter has examined the advantage of tailored information via IT, alongside designing resources for the Internet.
- Additional sections have highlighted the role of the health promoter in Internet advocacy and the move to reduce the digital divide.

ADDITIONAL READING

For more information on other aspects of IT not covered here, telemedicine, patient records and other medical systems, try Lenaghan, J (ed.) (1998) *Rethinking IT and health*. Institute for Public Policy Research, London.

For those interested in using the Internet in health promotion, this textbook covers the wide area of Internet health promotion: Rice, R E and Katz, J E (eds) (2001) *The Internet and health communication: experiences and expectations*. Sage, London.

For practitioners that want up-to-date information, regular reading of health promotion journal articles is recommended.

Using settings to communicate health promotion

Nova Corcoran and Anthony Bone

Learning objectives:

- Explore the features, roles and opportunities for the use of a settings-based approach in health promotion.
- Identify disadvantages and problems associated with a settings-based approach and consider ways to overcome these.
- Examine four non-traditional settings-based approaches and their potential to promote health.

The settings approach is not a new concept in health promotion. Increasing challenges to the promotion of health and the desire to ensure that health promotion is inclusive make debates around which settings to use and how to use them essential. Healthy settings embody the holistic notion of health promotion, as settings recognize that there are wider determinants that can impact on health. People obtain health information from a variety of sources beyond the doctor's surgery, as was shown in Choosing health: making healthy choices easier *(DOH 2004). These include friends and family and stories in newspapers and television, but this still represents a limited selection of sources. Clearly, sources of health information need to increase and people need to access a wider range of sources for their health needs. This chapter will examine the role of a settings-based approach, highlighting the different contexts that can be used. Four non-traditional settings have been chosen in this chapter for this purpose.*

DEFINING SETTINGS

Settings have received attention in policy documentation at national and international level. The philosophy of healthy settings stems from the *Ottawa Charter for Health Promotion* (WHO 1986), which emphasized not only the holistic notion of health – that 'health is created and lived by people within the settings of their everyday life; where they learn, work, play and love' (WHO 1986) – but also the role of healthy environments. This documentation served to highlight the role of settings as a framework where health can be created, promoted and improved in the context of daily lives and routines. The Charter additionally highlights that the responsibility for health promotion should be shared among the community and those who reside in them: individuals, community groups, health professionals, health service institutions and governments.

There are a wide range of settings that can be used in health promotion. One of the first was the worldwide concept of 'healthy cities' that links global initiatives with local action (WHO 2003). The city can be an appropriate setting to address factors that contribute to the health of different groups. This includes issues around poverty, pollution, sustainable development and social exclusion as well as the support received for health alliances, for example, between public, private and voluntary services.

In the UK the *Health of the nation* (DOH 1992) government document included the suitability of health promotion in schools, workplaces and hospitals. The document that replaced this, *Saving lives: our healthier nation* (DOH 1999), identified three settings, 'healthy schools, healthy workplaces and healthy neighbourhoods', as locations to address *inequalities* and promote health. The current UK government policy document *Choosing health: making healthy choices easier* (DOH 2004) continues to highlight the role of settings in the promotion of health in schools, communities and workplaces. The White Paper comments that 'the Government has a role in fostering demand for health, working with public services, the voluntary sector and industry to get accurate information and choices to people in ways that are relevant to their lives and meet their needs as individuals' (DOH 2004: 20).

The new UK government document *Our health, our care, our say: a new direction for community services* (DOH 2006a) further emphasizes the need for local health settings to promote health through its proposal to 'aim to provide more care in more local, convenient settings' (DOH 2006a: 9). The document indicates that more services will be delivered via settings, particularly those closer to home offering more choice to individuals. Sexual health, for example, is highlighted as an appropriate topic to promote through local settings, as delivery through hospital-based services is not appropriate or economic, and sexual health services are suitable for delivery through a range of settings.

The settings approach marks a move away from traditional health education to the promotion of holistic health, and has its roots embedded in new public health (Dooris and Thompson 2001). The move to integrate health promotion and public health together has led to a 'broader investment in structures that lay outside of traditional health service sectors' (Whitehead 2004) and marks a move away from individual health education towards holistic health promotion. The World Health Organisation indicate that settings themselves represent 'practical networks and projects to create healthy environments such as healthy schools, health-promoting hospitals, healthy workplaces and healthy cities' (WHO 1998: 1).

Activity 6.1:   Types of settings for different target groups

Think of a target group that might benefit from a health promotion intervention.

1   What sort of setting could be used to pass a health message to them?
2   What sort of restrictions could there be on giving a successful health message to this group?

TYPES OF SETTINGS

It has been postulated that a settings approach includes three aspects: a healthy living and working environment, integration of health promotion into daily activities, and links with the local community (Baric 1993). Dooris (2005) indicates that there is no clear consensus of a settings approach, although does propose that it is clear that settings share a number of important characteristics. First, health is seen as being determined by the wider environment. All settings take a broad definition of health whereby individual health is influenced by wider structures of health, rather than a biomedical, narrow definition of health. Second, the setting itself is a complex system of 'inputs, throughputs, outputs and impacts' (Dooris 2005: 56). Health therefore is part of the wider 'whole' of what an organization is trying to achieve, be it education, production of a product or financial gain. It is essential to remember that a setting is not a discrete entity, as there are wider factors that can influence a setting in the broader context of society. Third, organizational change and development is important, as for a true settings approach to be taken the organization often has to evolve or develop to achieve a healthy setting status.

Tones and Green (2004) distinguish between two different types of settings approaches in health promotion. The first approach is health promotion 'in a setting', for example, delivery of an intervention to increase uptake of screening. The second approach is 'using a setting' as a health promotion approach. This takes more of a comprehensive agenda and the setting is utilized in a wider health promotion sphere where environment, policy, interventions or target groups in that setting become part of the whole approach.

Settings allow health promotion to be practiced across a broad spectrum and can address the 'whole' problem rather than isolated parts (Whitelaw et al. 2001). This has the advantage of tackling health issues from a holistic angle. Another key feature of settings is that 'all activities are mutually supportive and combine synergistically to improve the health and well being of those who live or work or receive care there' (Tones and Green 2004: 270). Coordination and interaction are at the forefront of a successful setting.

Current ideas in the field of health promotion indicate that a settings approach is not just a delivery mechanism for health promotion as often utilized in the past. A settings approach takes a more holistic approach, incorporating the wider interactions of social, political and cultural movements and influences. Organizations and those who operate within their frameworks are going to be influenced by these variables. The settings approach can only be truly success-ful therefore when it moves to modifying contexts (social, political, environmen-tal, structural) rather than modifying individuals to improve health. This approach is sometimes referred to as the 'ecological approach' and allows the wider influences of health to be considered in totality. It has been further sug-gested that developing health policies and an evidence base should also be part of a settings approach (Naidoo and Wills 2000).

MAIN FEATURES OF SETTINGS

Whitelaw et al. (2001) propose five broad approaches to settings: the passive model, the active model, the vehicle model, the organic model and the compre-hensive model (see Figure 6.1).

These five broad approaches can be adopted by the practitioner depending on what is trying to be achieved. Small-scale interventions that aim to raise aware-ness of a health issue may be part of the passive model. Groups to encourage stopping smoking in a business that are partly supported by the organization might be part of the active model. Rewriting policies or plans for organizational changes in a supermarket might be part of the vehicle model. Training all staff in the correct use of a VDU (visual display unit, i.e. a computer monitor) might be part of the organic model. Finally, the comprehensive model includes inter-ventions that incorporate wider aspects of health, with organizational changes in policy or practice alongside possible investment or other features that aim to cre-ate a healthy 'whole' school or other 'whole' organization.

Activity 6.2:   Fitting activities to setting-based models

Using the examples in Figure 6.1 to help you decide which setting-based 'model' best fits these activities:

1   Staff training to increase knowledge of discrimination policies.
2   Anti-bullying strategy in a hospital.
3   Staff training for serving intoxicated customers in a pub with new licensing laws.
4   Healthy cities projects.
5   Cookery classes using low-fat foods.

Models	Setting approach	Brief description	Example
Passive	Neutral setting	Setting offers access to the population and a situation to conduct individual focussed activity	Intervention to raise knowledge of World Aids Day via an information stand
Active	Individual focussed	Individual focussed interventions but includes recognition of wider organization	Stop smoking programme in an organization where Nicotine Replacement Therapy is supplied by the organisation
Vehicle	Individual focussed + wider context	Setting is the problem, and individual projects can address these	No-smoking policies in a supermarket
Organic	Wider context	Setting is seen as the problem, but individual change is the solution	Office worker seminars for correct use of VDUs
Comprehensive	Entire context	Changing structures or cultures on a large scale via investment, policy, planning, laws, financial	Healthy schools programmes which include a holistic notion of health via changing structures

Figure 6.1   Settings-based models for health promotion, based on Whitelaw et al.'s (2001) model definitions

It has been argued that for the potential of a full settings approach to be achieved, only the last model (the comprehensive model) fulfils the full holistic criteria. However, given scarce resources, limited budgets, lack of time, expertise and a limited evidence base, the comprehensive model is often unachievable and unrealistic. Therefore this chapter will include the range of these five models as the other settings approaches continue to be implemented and practiced in health promotion work.

TRADITIONAL SETTINGS

Given the emphasis on policy and settings, some of the first references to settings were healthy hospitals, schools and workplaces (DOH 1992), thereby much of the literature focuses on these traditional settings (see additional reading at the end of this chapter). Traditional settings include those settings that are more widely used and can provide access to a sometimes easy-to-reach population. These include education venues such as schools, workplaces and health care services. For example, Bensberg and Kennedy (2002) advocate emergency departments as a setting for health promotion interventions. They are seen as an effective setting because they share similar goals to health promotion (for example, improving health), they are credible health information sources, utilize existing infrastructures for health promotion such as alliances, networks or planning, and are a point of entry into the health system. They are in a position to provide patient information, prevention strategies and make use of mass media interventions (especially safety or injury prevention). The hospital is also part of the wider community.

Activity 6.3:   Traditional and non-traditional settings

1 Think of as many settings that can be used for health promotion as you can (large and small).
2 Which of these do you think are traditional settings and which are non–traditional settings?

One area where healthy settings have developed dramatically is in the 'health schools' movement. In the UK, Healthy Schools programmes are now overseen by the National Healthy Schools Programme (NHSP). Schools are encouraged to apply for health school status based on national quality standards. Government documentation proposed that half of all schools will be healthy schools by 2006, with the rest working towards healthy school status by 2009 (DOH 2004). Recent government policy along these lines has been directed at schools with the 'Healthy living blueprint for school' (DfES 2004b) that *supports children in leading a healthy lifestyle and makes the most of the resources that already exist*, encouraging schools to play a more active part in shaping attitudes to health and encouraging informed choice.

NON-TRADITIONAL SETTINGS

Tones and Green (2004) argue that if a settings approach is to avoid reaching those who are already in a more privileged position, for example those who are employed or in schools, different settings should be considered in order to avoid increasing the gap between the richest and poorest groups. For example, an intervention aimed at those in schools will not reach those excluded from school, and interventions in workplaces will exclude those who are unemployed. They propose that settings will 'need to address the needs of marginalized groups and include … unconventional and challenging settings' (Tones and Green 2004: 271). This means choosing settings for health promotion that are not traditionally used.

Non-traditional settings refer to settings that have not been frequently used in health promotion. These settings have hard-to-reach populations, use unusual methods or locations, and may be one-off. More unusual settings have been used in health promotion over time, for example 'healthy farms' (Thurston et al. 2005). Other settings have been used where non-traditional populations can be located, for example 'healthy prisons' (DOH 2002).

THE ADVANTAGES OF USING SETTINGS

There are a number of advantages to a settings approach in general. Dooris (2005) lists a number of these, which include providing a framework to utilize in practice, allowing ownership of health, enabling relationship exploration, recognition of existing initiatives, joined-up working and an awareness of health at all levels. The very nature of settings encourages multi-disciplinary and joint working to achieve objectives. The other advantage of settings is the 'normalization' of aspects of health. For example, if sexual health information was given to everyone in a workplace and discussed in a more open context, this may encourage a growing dialogue of discussion and encourage more people to access sexual health services when needed.

There are a number of aspects of the *settings-based approach* that are common to all settings and foster positive steps in health promotion. Peterson et al. (2002) proposes seven elements found to be beneficial to establishing church-based health promotion programmes (see Figure 6.2). Peterson proposes that a strong church-based programme will contain: 'partnerships, positive health values, availability of services, access to facilities, community-focussed interventions, healthy behaviour change, and supportive relationships' (Peterson et al. 2002: 403). Given the broad nature of these seven elements and the nature of the church as an institution, it is equally likely that these seven elements can be applied to other settings, with emphasis on their importance fluctuating depending upon the nature of the setting.

'Partnerships' include collaboration between organizations or the local community, particularly important for sustainability and involvement of key decision makers. 'Positive health values' include the well-known variables of health promotion practice: advocating, enabling and mediating. These three variables need to be engaged to promote health holistically. 'Availability of services' and 'Access to facilities' are needed to enable access to resources that are needed in the promotion of health, for example, money, equipment or other spaces. 'Community focussed' includes the value of the wider community, who when included will be able to assist in providing access and availability to resources. 'Health behaviour change' should include a focus on theory to support any behaviour changes, and 'social support' should be available via networks or groups for supporting change.

Element	Description
Partnerships	Collective collaboration between organization and other sectors (e.g. church and health professionals, supermarkets, wider community groups)
Positive health values	Advocate, enable, mediate, service, caring Promote, prevent, education to obtain positive health Use of organization for peer education to take an active role in health
Availability of services	Wider access to services or increased access to services, across potentially varied populations
Access to facilities	Resources available in the setting (e.g. meeting places, kitchen, exercise spaces) with the needed volunteers
Community focussed	Settings should value and include wider community (e.g. volunteers from community)
Health behaviour change	Theoretical concepts are important; desire to change unhealthy behaviours should be included in the setting and supported (e.g. fruit and vegetables at functions and support)
Social systems support	Social systems support in the setting and in wider community networks (e.g. the surrounding community, schools, offices); the networks should provide support for change

Figure 6.2   The seven key elements beneficial to establishing programmes, based on Peterson et al.'s (2002) elements for church-based health promotion programs

THE DISADVANTAGES OF USING SETTINGS

Currently the settings approach has a limited evidence base (Dooris 2005), although some areas are more popular than others, with the use of schools in particular attracting a growing evidence base. What should be of consideration in settings are groups who are excluded from that setting. Some settings have limited potential or contain alienated or disadvantaged groups who are resistant to interventions (Tones and Green 2004), and the development of non-traditional settings merits attention.

Settings can be individualistic, exclusive and have practical limitations (Tones and Green 2004). Health promotion in a settings context should involve everyone in the wider planning process. A settings approach that is centred on a 'top-down' approach tends to be ineffective (Whitelaw et al. 2001). When one (or a small number) of people dictate what will happen, it will be less effective than involving everyone in that setting. Settings that embody this 'top-down' approach neglect the wider context of the setting and will be more likely to exclude or alienate groups. Limited planning, lack of theoretical foundations and poor evaluation mean that interventions will be unsustainable (Bensberg and Kennedy 2002) and if left unevaluated or poorly evaluated, positive outcomes that have been achieved will never be recognized.

There are a number of practical limitations to a settings approach. These include finance, resources, time, location, manpower or other aspects that influence settings activities. For example, larger, private organizations may have more financial support than smaller, public ones. There will also be other competing priorities which mitigate against health priorities. The aim of an organization is not necessarily in line with the fundamental goals of health promotion. If an organization is concerned with speeding up the production of a product to make more money and the planned intervention requires finance or proposes changes that slow down the production process, health promotion will have to compete with these priorities. The outcome therefore might be that only part of the proposed changes take place, if any at all.

A settings-based approach is not going to be favourable to all concerned, particularly if it requires finances, resources or changes which can be difficult, such as structural changes. The settings that tend to incorporate a health promotion framework are more likely to be those that are better set up to deliver and involve others in health promotion – hence schools are a prime example, as few people can argue about the merit of promoting health of children, and often strong parental or teacher involvement can facilitate the health promotion process.

Whitelaw et al. (2001) argue that problems in the settings-based approach includes practitioners undertaking health promotion work with little focus or understanding of working within an organization but continue to use the label of a setting-based approach. This often has the effect of continuing a limited individualistic approach, which can lead to victim-blaming, alongside the role of the organization in health promotion being ignored. The wider environment needs consideration to avoid victim-blaming approaches (Bensberg and Kennedy 2002).

Activity 6.4:   Overcoming disadvantages of settings

Read the 'disadvantages' section of Chapter 6.

1   How do you think you could overcome some of these disadvantages if you were using a workplace setting to promote health?

OVERVIEW OF FOUR NON-TRADITIONAL SETTINGS

The four non-traditional settings that will be examined are: places of worship, universities, personal care (barbers, hairdressers and beauty salons) and travel centres. The first two have a reasonably strong evidence base supporting their role as an appropriate setting for health promotion. The second two have an evidence base predominately made up of 'grey' literature, which makes them more challenging. This is not to say that more challenging settings should be ignored in favour of easier settings; if health promotion is to be truly holistic, then more difficult settings will need to start becoming involved in the settings-based movement.

PLACES OF WORSHIP

Opportunities and advantages

Religious organizations and faith groups have often been able to engage in important roles in health (Duan et al. 2005) and thus have potential as a health promotion setting. They can provide a 'promising opportunity to enhance emotional, physical and spiritual health' (Peterson et al. 2002: 401) and 'faith and spiritual beliefs play a role in maintaining health and wellbeing' (Swinney et al. 2001: 42). The role of religious organizations fits with a holistic definition of health, including physical and emotional aspects of health, alongside spiritual aspects of health and the role of a healthy body, mind, soul and spirit which are integral to religious organizations (Peterson et al. 2002).

Most research has focussed on Christian churches, and has demonstrated that the church is a potentially effective channel for the delivery of health promotion programmes (Resnicow et al. 2002) as well as conclusions that suggest that church attendance correlates with positive health care practices and preventative behaviours (Aaron et al. 2003; Benjamins and Brown 2004). Advantages can include a strong social support role (Duan et al. 2005) in addition to a tendency to respond to the needs of its community. Religious organizations can influence the health of its members, for example, Swinney et al. (2001) found that church parishioners believed the church has a role in meeting health needs of its congregation, suggesting there is some expectation that the church will fulfil this role. Markens et al. (2002), in their interviews with pastors of black churches, suggest that pastors also saw health as something that should be promoted through their work in the church community. Therefore the Christian church may be a place where health promotion could take place where both religious leaders and the religious community may be willing to attend and participate. In 1995 a report in Derby in the UK found that religious organizations were actively undertaking activities that can be classed as health promotion (Andrews et al. 1995). These included assertiveness and defence classes for women, keep fit and health seminars, education classes for children, leisure activities for young and older people as well as other health-related activities.

The advantages of using religious organizations in health promotion are wide-ranging and may allow access to some sub-populations (Duan et al. 2005), including ethnic groups, older people and women, who may be traditionally low-users of health care services. Another advantage is that religious organizations are distributed throughout countries (Duan et al. 2005), where they can include whole populations or sections of the population who attend a religious organization. These organizations have a tradition as being a strong caring foundation (Peterson et al. 2002) providing financial, emotional or spiritual support in times of need. This also gives them the benefit of being a place where social support networks exist. Peterson et al. (2002) highlight the role of social support in the adoption of healthy behaviours, drawing attention to women's adoption of physical activity being more likely with social support. A focus on spiritual health may also provide a motivating factor for change (Peterson et al. 2002). Alongside social support, religious organizations can provide a social life (Christensen et al. 2005) for parishioners, with sermons, mid-week classes, Sunday schools, outings or fundraisers as wider aspects of church attendance. As an actual setting a religious organization can provide a safe, supportive environment (Peterson et al. 2002), which can help facilitate behaviour changes.

Role models and credible sources of information in religious organizations include religious leaders. Leaders of these organizations tend to be demographically similar to members, and embody values similar to their congregations (Reinert et al. 2003); it is also likely that given that membership is voluntary, the leaders chosen are viewed as trustworthy sources of information, making them more likely role models.

Recently, places of religious organizations have been used for health promotion and health education interventions in a variety of ways, but most commonly to change individual behaviours in relation to lifestyle-related behaviours. Renicow et al. (2001) undertook an 'eat for life' project in an African American group, and found an increase in fruit and vegetable consumption. Duan et al. (2005) found an increase in mammography uptake after a project to encourage mammography screening uptake. Campbell et al. (2004) undertook the 'WATCH' intervention to encourage colectoral cancer preventive behaviours, which was met with some success as it improved behaviours (for example, fruit and vegetable consumption) which can lower colectoral cancer risks. 'Project DIRECT' aimed to decrease the burden of diabetes in relation to self-management of diabetes, exercise and diet (Reid et al. 2003). Other projects have utilized health workers in the actual setting.

Implications for practice

Lewis et al. (2000) suggest the use of theories and models, and to design programmes that are effective and not duplicating programmes that groups do not want. The Peterson et al.'s (2002) framework described earlier (Figure 6.2), which highlights partnerships, positive health values, availability of services, access to facilities, community-focussed interventions, healthy behaviour change and supportive relationships, was originally designed for a church setting. Therefore any intervention that utilizes this setting could use this framework as a starting point for a settings-based programme designed to promote effective behaviour change. Other research suggests the use of parishioners as role models or educators. Duan et al. (2005) used female parishioners as peer counsellors to promote mammography and adherence. Another potential motivating factor is the inclusion of religious and spiritual themes into health promotion messages (see Case Study 6.1).

Case Study 6.1   Healthy body health spirit

Resnicow et al. (2002), in their study 'Healthy body/Healthy Spirit', targeted African Americans, and the intervention materials involved the parishioners in their design. They used biblical and spiritual message to reinforce motivation. The design of an 'eat for life' cookbook included recipes submitted by the church group. Other resources followed a spiritual and religious theme. For example, videos included biblical and spiritual themes to motivate healthy eating and an audio cassette designed for performing exercise to gospel music combined with spiritual messages to match the length of the workout routine.

Activity 6.5:   Designing messages for a religious group

1   Choose a religious group.
2   Based on the ideas in Case Study 6.1, what other resources could be designed to promote health using a biblical or spiritual message in a religious group?

Religious organizations with strong leadership roles are more likely to sustain projects in the long term. Research suggests longevity of the church indicates sustainability of projects, as does the active membership size (Duan et al. 2005). Christensen et al. (2005) found that religious organizations with stable, consistent leadership are the most likely to express interest in a health-related programme for cancer prevention, and competing priorities were the most likely reasons for refusal. They also found that smaller organizations were the most interested in a cancer prevention programme, suggesting perhaps less competing priorities.

Points to consider

There are gaps in the literature on religious organizations and their role in public health (Christensen et al. 2005). There is a distinct African-American US focus in many studies, leaving other groups missing from the research (Christensen et al. 2005; Peterson et al. 2002). A limited evidence base for health promotion and health education work utilizing other faith groups means that other religious groups, such as Muslim or Sheik groups, are not evident in the research. This has some implications for research, given that it is unclear whether different places of worship – mosques or temples, for example – are appropriate settings to promote health. Poor dissemination of results and few controlled designs also means that the evidence base remains patchy (Peterson et al. 2002).

Despite barriers, church-based health promotion interventions still hold promise for accessing diverse populations (Peterson et al. 2002) and is an under-utilized settings for the promotion of health on a small and large scale. If health promotion is truly to achieve health for all, and access some of the harder-to-reach groups, particularly older age groups, women and some ethnic minority groups, a variety of religious organizations will need to be included within health promotion frameworks.

UNIVERSITIES

Opportunities and advantages

Universities have a key role to play in the promotion of health of those working and studying within their walls and to the wider community. It has been proposed that universities face a number of challenges in the 20th century, including higher delivery expectation, quality, demographic changes and higher costs (Comm and Mathaisel, 2003), meaning that universities face dilemmas of re-structuring to enable institutions to become better and more efficient than before.

Universities were not originally included in the first concepts of the 'settings' approaches to health (Whitehead 2004; Dooris 2001) and consequently have not been at the forefront of the settings approach to health. There is a lack of international or national standards around health promoting universities, although the UK government document *Choosing health: making health choices easier* (DOH 2004) does highlight the importance of integrating health into the organizational structures of universities and colleges. The WHO (1998) published a working document on health promoting universities highlighting that 'the settings-based approach to health promotion can potentially enhance the contribution of universities to improving the health of populations' (Tsouros et al. 1998: 3).

Those health promoting universities that do exist have often adopted a student-centred approach (rather than staff). Health promotion campaigns involving students, via the student union for example, are most commonly used (Dunne and Somerset 2004), and less attention has been given to staff or the move to a 'whole' university approach. The student union remains an obvious choice for health promotion work. They are in close contact with the health needs of its members because they are elected and are drawn from the client population so the needs are known at first hand. The health agenda is also appropriate to settings; for example, advice about the stresses of student life including financial, welfare, sexual health and other health-related topics.

Although whole university approaches have been slow in coming, there are few reasons why universities should not be key health promotion settings. They share similar characteristics with other educational facilities, for example schools and workplaces, both of which are highlighted as appropriate health promotion settings (DOH 2004). Universities tend to be large organizations employing a variety of staff (academic and non-academic, technical, researcher and others) and are in a good position to promote health of students (Dunne and Somerset 2004) and staff. Dooris and Thompson (2001) consider that universities are well placed for a settings-based approach to health promotion for a number of reasons, including: their focus on education, training and research, a role in developing and creating innovation, and the fact that universities are a community resource. The university is also a setting where skills can be taught in a safe, supportive environment (Xiangyang et al. 2003), making it ideally placed for a healthy setting.

Case Study 6.2   University of Central Lancashire

The University of Central Lancashire is one of the first and only UK-based universities to embody the health promotion settings approach. The health university initiative aims 'to integrate within the university's culture, processes and structures a commitment to health and to developing its health promoting potential land to promote the health and well-being of staff, students and the wider community' (UCLAN 2006). To achieve this, a variety of initiatives have been put into place in the university setting. These include new policies (corporate health policy and transport policies), student and staff health-related information (health handbooks, sexual health projects) and changes in the curriculum and research to encourage health into other non-health disciplines.

(UCLAN 2006)

Implications for practice

'One of the most valuable roles for a health promoting university … is … to become an advocate for developing healthy public policy at both local and national level' (Dooris and Thompson 2001: 159). Davis et al. (2003) suggest higher education could be an important leader or model for adopting pro-sustainability behaviours and policies.

Xiangyang et al. (2003) propose a five-stage framework that can be used to adopt a healthy university setting. Figure 6.3 illustrates the five stages that a university will need to consider before becoming a health promotion university. 'Adopting' includes the adoption and revision of current policies in the university that currently support or hinder health promotion. 'Creating' includes the creation of supportive environments. This can include anything from health and safety policies to the provision of bicycle lock-up areas. 'Developing' includes the development of personal skills, for example, coping skills or self-esteem.

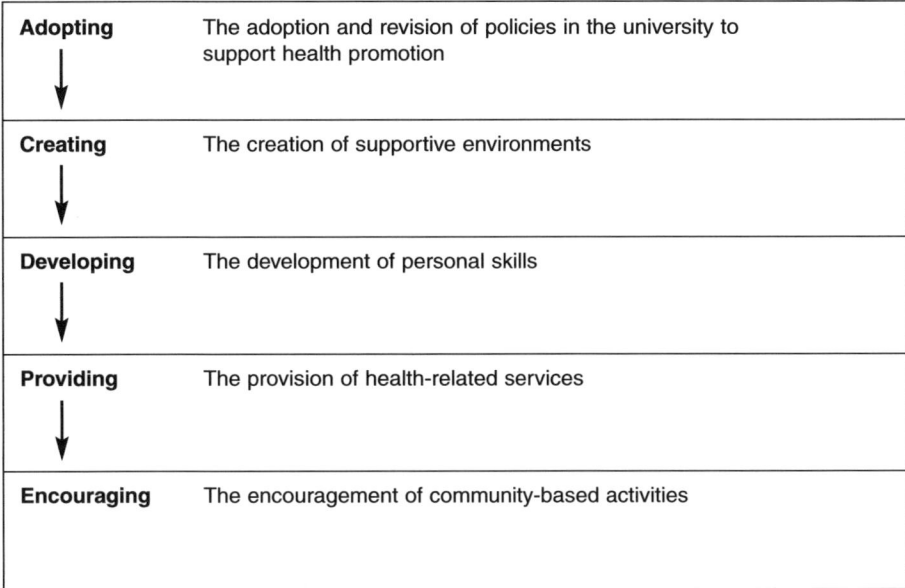

Adopting	The adoption and revision of policies in the university to support health promotion
Creating	The creation of supportive environments
Developing	The development of personal skills
Providing	The provision of health-related services
Encouraging	The encouragement of community-based activities

Figure 6.3   Five-stage framework for healthy universities, adapted from Xiangyang et al. (2003)

'Providing' include the provision of health-related services. This could include smoking cessation services, counselling services or even fitness clubs. 'Encouraging' includes engaging the wider community to become a partner in the project. Students and staff should have links with the wider community and vice versa to enable sustainability of projects.

Activity 6.6:   Designing healthy university resources

View the on-line poster for 'Healthy living blueprint for schools' (DfES 2004a) through the website www.publications.teachernet.gov.uk.

1   Using the ideas in this poster, what design features would you decide to have for a poster for a university health campaign to promote better diet and nutrition in students?
2   What advantages does a university have in functioning as a health setting?

Points to consider

Dooris and Thompson (2001) highlight a number of challenges to a health promoting university. These include organization, ownership and different setting perspectives. Organization can be difficult, for example, where to locate the project(s). If it is to include the whole university a student/staff split should not be evident, which makes it more difficult to choose the location. Implementation depends on cooperation, both internal and external (Xiangyang et al. 2003). Project ownership is another challenge; for example, the whole university should be involved in managing and working towards sustainability, although this may be difficult to achieve without initial leadership. A different settings perspective may be shared by different staff and students. Potentially controversial topics such as workloads or working conditions may be considered inappropriate, yet if the university is to take a wide settings approach these topics will need to be included in an initial address. Evaluation also needs to be added to the planning process. Long-term measurement can be difficult, especially if different cohorts of students are being measured. Full-time students traditionally take three or four years to complete their programmes, and measurement may involve another cohort, making generalizations difficult.

Universities have the capacity to change and a 'responsibility to educate and influence the next generation of decision makers and managers' (Dooris and Thompson 2001: 106). The university setting is gaining recognition as a potentially effective setting to promote health (Dunne and Somerset 2004). It is hoped that policy support such as *Choosing health: making healthy choices easier* (DOH 2004) will help translate words into action. Healthy universities need to evolve in their creation of national and international standards to enable all the good work achieved by 'healthy schools' to continue into adulthood education.

PERSONAL CARE SETTINGS

Opportunities and advantages

Disappointingly, the evidence base is not widely available for the use of beauty salons, barbers and hairdressers as a setting for health promotion. This is not due to lack of projects in these areas, rather that there are a number of small-scale projects ongoing that are not incorporated into the evidence base, and the available evidence can mostly be found in research that makes up the body of grey literature. There is some support for these settings; the Department of Health (2003), for example, recognizes that hairdressers have a role to play in sexual health promotion and health education projects (DOH 2003). A variety of health promotion departments worldwide have been using salons, barber shops and hairdressers to promote health. An example is Thameside Sexual Health Services in the UK, which describe a community initiative that trained 12 local women's hairdressers around sexual health, gave a supply of condoms (displayed on the counter, for example) and information about sexual health services to enable them to engage in conversations around sexual health (Johnstone 1999). Lewis et al. (2002) also report on the Barber and Beautician STD/HIV Peer Educator Programme, where local barbers and beauticians educated clients about STDs (now STIs) and HIV and distributed condoms and educational materials.

Activity 6.7:   Using barbers or beauty salons

Choose either barbers or beauty salons as a setting.

1   What sort of health promotion topics could be covered in this setting?
2   What are the disadvantages of using this setting? How might you overcome these?

Given the nature of other personal care settings, these settings could have potential to deliver interventions at a wider level. Linnan et al. (2001) propose four levels – intrapersonal, interpersonal, organizational and community – which could be delivered via the beauty salon (and similar) settings (see Figure 6.4). Interventions on an intrapersonal level could include publicity material available at the reception desk or waiting areas. Interpersonal level interventions could be discussions with the client instigated by the provider around health issues. Organizational interventions include using wider aspects of the settings, for example, introducing policies designed to promote health to the whole salon or studio environment. Community-based interventions include those which involve the wider community, for example, the setting becoming an educational resource for the whole community.

Intrapersonal	Publicity material with health messages including leaflets, posters, flyers, videos or information booklets
Interpersonal	Interaction between more than one person (e.g. client and care provider) including discussion, one-to-one or question/answer
Organizational	Policies or interventions on a wider scale in the salon setting (e.g. healthy food or drinks for clients or no-smoking policies)
Community	Involving community in design or implementation of an intervention (e.g. becoming an education resource for the whole community, being involved in whole community activities)

Figure 6.4   The multi-level interventions in a personal care setting

The North Carolina 'BEAUTY and Health' pilot study (Linnan et al. 2005) indicated that cosmetologists delivered cancer prevention messages around a number of cancer-related key topics (designed in conjunction with the stakeholders in the programme). The cosmetologists continued to deliver these messages up to 12 months after the pilot intervention, with more than half of the customers reported to have visited their health care providers since the study, indicating the feasibility of cosmetologists and beauty salon owners in the health promotion delivery interventions.

Beauty salons have the advantage of being women focussed, with frequent attendees. A reasonable time period is spent there (30 minutes upwards), where a wide range of topics are discussed between client and cosmetologist (Linnan et al. 2001). One important topic to focus on is the link between beauty and health (Linnan et al. 2001), and the salon environment is already set to discuss these issues (Linnan et al. 2005). Women attend beauty salons with a motivation to look attractive or beautiful, therefore health promotion plays an important role in achieving this goal. Solomon et al. (2004) also propose that the social environment in a beauty salon encourages conversation, information-giving and advice, with several conversations leading to health topics, and often there are displays in salons that promote healthy messages, for example healthy eating. The salon setting is a feasible and desirable setting to introduce health promotion messages, given the health topics that cosmetologists say they discuss with their clients (Linnan et al. 2005). For example, eating fresh fruit and vegetables with their vitamin and mineral properties are linked to strong nails and good hair quality.

Barber shops have always been traditionally male-dominated environments. Barbers are a location where men gather to enjoy company and can be sources of entertainment or conversation, including facilities such as television, games or videos (Lewis et al. 2002). This indicates that time may be divided between self-care and leisure. There is evidence to suggest that there are successful small-scale initiatives which use barber shops. These schemes have targeted a mixture of ethnic minority groups, for example, the 'Health of Men' project in Bradford and Airedale is aimed at targeting men from Asian communities and aims to break down barriers and cross cultural boundaries to empower men to look after their health more effectively (Men's Health Forum 2004).

Case Study 6.3   Wolverhampton PCT barber shop scheme

The barber shop scheme in Wolverhampton ran from 1998 to 2003 in 12 barber shops. The scheme aimed to increase condom usage among the African Caribbean community and increase access to health information. A questionnaire evaluation indicated that the scheme reduced embarrassment, possibly through the social environment delivery methods. Evaluation also indicated that the scheme raised awareness and provided education on STIs through the promotion of safer sex.

Points to consider

There are a number of creative programmes utilizing beauty salons, but few are evaluated (Linnan et al. 2001). The evidence base for using personal care settings is limited, despite the potential role of these locations to promote health. The grey literature has projects that run worldwide, but disappointingly practitioners are not making these projects readily accessible for others. Future practice should aim to undertake well-planned campaigns in these settings, with clear evaluation frameworks to encourage best practice.

Not all topics are suitable for these 'open' and sociable environments, and some clients may not consider it appropriate to discuss some health topics, especially more sensitive subjects. However, it is clear that some topics, such as healthy eating, sensible drinking or stopping smoking, have a role to play in appearance and could be good topics for this setting. The salon or studio environment is accessed by a range of clients and customers who should be included in the design of projects to enable their future success.

TRAVEL CENTRES

Opportunities and advantages

It is recognized that while on holiday people may put themselves in more risky situations, for example, unsafe sex or drinking too much alcohol. Other risks include exposure to different illnesses or diseases. A report by the National Public Health Service for Wales (2005) examined impacts of UK tourism and health and found that risk behaviour increases on holiday, especially in relation to alcohol or drug misuse and sexual behaviours. Another suggestion was that a number of visits to health care services by tourists could be prevented by pre-travel preventive care.

Provost et al. (2002) found that travel agents recommendations are important in influencing travellers to seek preventive advice alongside the fact that travel agents are in a good position to encourage travellers to consult travel clinics. There is also some evidence to suggest there are reasonably high levels of recall of advice from travel clinics (Bauer 2002). Travel agents have been involved in some small-scale projects, for example NHS Scotland (2003) runs an annual media campaign to address heterosexual transmission of HIV via holiday packs that are available at a variety of locations including travel agents.

The convenience of this setting for health care delivery must not be overlooked, and this is an excellent setting from an opportunistic health context. Most travel agents believed they had a role in the prevention of health problems in travellers, especially in consulting a travel clinic (Provost et al. 2002). Thus while users may well be aware of mechanical requirements for travel, for example immunisation, there is also the opportunity to give more general advice to protect the travellers health. Examples could be health advice for the travelling process, such as prevention of deep vein thrombosis (DVT) in air travel. Health while on holiday could also be included. Sun safety, alcohol, sexual health, illegal drugs or theft are all areas where the holidaymaker could receive important preventive advice.

There is also a role in travel health for more traditional health information for travel to high-risk areas. Duval (2003) found that travellers were more likely to visit a travel clinic if they fell into a high-risk area. The traveller can be made aware that ill health may result from their holiday environment (at least in certain countries). Van Herck et al. (2003) found that around one-third of travellers questioned had not sought pre-travel health advice, and only a minority were vaccinated as per current recommendations. Wilder-Smith (2003) found similar numbers of travellers seeking pre-travel advice. This suggests that not only should travel agents be highlighting health prevention and risk information, and directing to appropriate locations or services if appropriate, but perhaps that airports, train stations or other places of travel should also play a role in providing this information, and it is surprising that this area has received little attention as a potential health promotion location.

One topic that has received some attention in travel centres is sexual health, or more accurately the prevention of STIs. Matteelli and Carosi (2001) indicate that although evidence suggests that travellers have an increased risk of acquiring STIs, prevention receives a low priority in travel clinics. The suggestion is that travellers with an increased risk should be targeted for interventions. The Health Protection Agency (2003) draws attention to the link between those taking sexual risks on holidays being more likely to take sexual health risks at home. They underline the importance of pro-active sexual health education prior to departure as part of the range of health messages given to travellers.

Activity 6.8:   Opportunistic settings use and travel health

As part of the three-year alcohol awareness campaign in Ireland from 2001, the design of an alcohol travel wallet announcement was created. The advertisement was designed to be displayed on travel tickets targeting young people with the slogan 'less is more' (Health Promotion Unit 2006).
    If you were designing a campaign to promote safety from theft when travelling:

1   What messages might you give to emphasize safety or risk?
2   What methods would you use to get your messages across to travellers? And where would you put these messages so they were seen?

Points to consider

There is no correct way to undertake opportunistic health promotion, apart from the fact it should reach those through an opportunity such as through a travel agent or an airport. Materials are less likely to have an opportunity to be tailored, but should still follow designs suggested in previous chapters. The production of information packs given to travellers might be a starting point, containing travel advice and help-lines, together with free condoms, first-aid kits or other health promotion materials. These could be distributed to travel agents to be passed to holidaymakers when they book their holidays or made available to travellers in airports or railway stations. Alternatively, the involvement of large airline companies in the design of materials could also be useful.

The suggestion of a development of, or access to, existing networks in public health to inform travel agents of prevention of traveller's health problems may be one way to ensure that travel agents and clinics have access to the information they need, and the support and resources they need, to be able to give health information opportunistically.

CONCLUSION

Dooris (2005) argues that there is still a lack of evidence base for a settings approach. This is partly due to the focus on single factors, for example one disease or risk, in the settings approach. He argues that the application of theoretical-based evidence to a setting approach is needed alongside decision makers who are engaged in the planning and evaluation levels (Chapter 7 considers *evidence-based practice* in more detail). When undertaking settings-based activities, the ◀◀ evidence base should be examined as thoroughly as possible, including the grey literature (see Chapter 7). Settings-based activities should also be based on clear expectations (Whitelaw et al. 2001). Using a setting may provide access to an entire community, but this is not to say that everyone in that community will want to be involved; finance, time, resources, disinterest are all obstacles which will need to be overcome or worked with. 'It is becoming increasingly clear that 21st century problems can only be meaningfully tackled through adopting holistic and comprehensive approaches within the places that people live their lives' (Dooris 2005: 63). Health promoters of today should be constantly seeking to adopt comprehensive approaches in tune with wider population needs.

Summary

- This chapter has highlighted the role of the settings-based approach in health promotion and has defined settings and their characteristics.
- This chapter has considered taking into consideration their advantages and disadvantages.
- This chapter has explored four non-traditional settings in health promotion. These include two large settings, religious organizations and universities, alongside two smaller settings, personal care and travel centres.
- The merits of these settings to promote health were highlighted together with their challenges to the promotion of health.

ADDITIONAL READING

For comprehensive coverage of a variety of settings including the health services, local authorities, workplaces and education settings, try Scriven, A and Orme, J (2001) *Health promotion professional perspectives*. Palgrave, Basingstoke.

An interesting chapter on the settings-based approach can also be found in Tones, K and Green, J (2004) *Health promotion: planning and strategies*. Sage, London.

The Health Settings Development Unit, part of the University of Central Lancashire, has some easily accessible information with links to many major settings policy documentation at www.uclan.ac.uk/facs/health/hsdu/index.htm

7

Evidence-based practice and communication

Nova Corcoran and John Garlick

Learning objectives:

- Explore the role of evidence-based practice in health promotion interventions.
- Examine the application of evidence to health promotion interventions via a number of mechanisms.
- Identify problematic areas of evidence-based practice and consider ways to overcome these.

Health promotion interventions now frequently use evidence-based practice to enhance the likelihood of successful outcomes, although this has not curbed the lively debate around evidence-based practice. The appropriateness of using evidence in health promotion, the types of evidence to use alongside the applicability and transferability of this evidence to practice are all sources of ongoing discussion. On the one hand, health practitioners are being continually reminded that evidence-based practice is important to health promotion and health education work, and there is a growing evidence base accordingly. On the other hand, they are being urged to exercise caution when applying the available evidence to their work. This chapter will examine what evidence can be used in health promotion, and the potential problems that can arise from utilizing the evidence base. Acceptability and transferability of evidence will be explored, alongside how to establish and use the evidence available in practical work.

DEFINITIONS OF EVIDENCE-BASED PRACTICE

The use of evidence in informing the development of health care practice is not new. Sackett et al. (1996) referred to the philosophical origins of evidence based medicine extending back to mid-19th century Paris and earlier. They noted that evidence based medicine, defined as the conscientious, explicit and judicious use of best evidence in making decisions about the care of individual patients, remained a hot topic amongst clinicians, public health practitioners, purchasers, planners and the public. Criticisms included that it was 'old hat', that it was aimed at cost-cutting and that it would suppress clinical freedom. Amidst this debate evidence based medicine continued to evolve and adapt. The principles of the evidence base movement were soon taken up in nursing, with DiCenso et al. (1998) defining evidence based nursing as the process by which nurses make clinical decisions, using the best available research evidence, their clinical expertise and patient preferences, in the context of available resources. Gray (2001) went further and took the concept of evidence based decision making in health beyond purely clinical practice and applied it to groups of patients, or populations, which might be manifested as evidence based policy-making, purchasing or management.

Evidence in health promotion and its use in practice has received a mixed reception, with arguments ranging from health promotion success being wholly reliant on demonstration of a strong evidence base, to arguments that suggest health promotion and evidence are incompatible (McQueen 2000). Arguments continue to persist. The 51st World Health Assembly urged all member states to 'adopt an evidence-based approach to health promotion policy and practice, using the full range of quantitative and qualitative methodologies' (WHA 1998). By contrast, McQueen noted that as recently as 1998 the word 'evidence' had no place in the World Health Organization Health Promotion Glossary (WHO 1998).

The premise of *Communicating health: strategies for health promotion* is that for health promotion to be successful there is a need to look at evidence critically and apply what works in order to demonstrate effectiveness. Given that health promotion has a variety of aims, this includes to justify decisions that have been made, to evaluate effectiveness or efficiency of an intervention, or to justify resources, time or funding.

An evidence based approach is one that 'incorporates into policy and practice decision processes and the findings from a critical examination of demonstrated intervention effects' (Rychetnik and Wise 2004: 248), or as proposed by Wiggers and Sanson-Fisher (2001), the systematic integration of evidence into the planning process of health promotion activities. Evidence-based practice is about making sure that an intervention is supported by evidence, enabling the design of a successful intervention (Harrison 2003). There are a number of different ways that the words 'evidence-based practice' have been used. In the area of public health, Harrison (2003) divides these into three categories, which can be adapted to health promotion practice (see Figure 7.1).

In health promotion practice, the practitioner will usually make use of 'the evidence base for public health' (or health promotion), to either make evidence-based policy and practice decisions or utilize the evidence to inform their own policy and practice.

---

1 **Evidence-based policy and practice**
   Practice that attempts to use current evidence to make a judgement or decision on the most appropriate intervention(s).
2 **Evidence-informed policy and practice**
   A situation where evidence (usually a wide range of evidence) has been used to inform an intervention.
3 **The evidence base for public health**
   This includes the whole catalogue of evidence available for public health interventions, policies or practice and can be used by practitioners to inform their practice.

Figure 7.1   Three categories of evidence-based practice

RATIONALE FOR EVIDENCE BASE

All practitioners, including those involved in policy design, development and management should be aware of the current evidence base (Rychetnik and Wise 2004). There is increasing recognition of the importance of evidence-based practice that can be used to justify health promotion activity (Tones and Green 2004) and an agreement that health promotion programmes 'should be based on clear and rigorous evidence about their efficacy' (Harrison 2003: 229).

The rationale for using the evidence base is strong. It has been argued that there is an ethical imperative to employ evidence so that health promotion does no harm (Tones and Green 2004). This theme is also taken up by Raphael, who argues that ethical health promotion practice requires clear recognition of the 'ideologies, values, principles and rules of evidence' (2000: 355). Another important reason is the move to close the gap between theory and practice, alongside increased confidence of practitioners that the decisions they have made are the correct ones. Tones and Green propose that 'systematic planning of health promotion requires a series of decisions to be made at each stage' (2004: 330) and that decisions should be based on the best available evidence at that time. Wang et al. (2005) also agree that evidence-based practice in public health should mean that health care decisions are based on the best evidence available.

Current ideas would suggest that unless multidisciplinary areas such as health promotion and public health utilize the evidence base, practitioners will continually have to defend decisions that have been made without evidence. Harrison argues that without evidence practitioners will be 'open to the charge that while its intentions are well meaning, its prescriptions require better demonstration of their effectiveness' (2003: 228). While other disciplines around health promotion are using evidence, for example medicine and physiotherapy, health promotion is in danger of becoming a discipline that cannot prove that interventions are cost-effective, reliable, valid or acceptable unless it starts and continues to incorporate elements of evidence-based practice into all areas of its discipline.

Activity 7.1:   Evidence-based practice rationale

1   Can you think of any other reasons why evidence-based practice might be important to health promotion practice?

Rychetnik and Wise (2004) propose two questions to consider when using an evidence base in health promotion. First, is the evidence relevant and useful to current policy and practice contexts, and second, what is the reviewer's role in a) interpretation and b) advocating action based on that interpretation? Tones and Green (2004) suggest that with evidence the question should go beyond the fundamental 'does it work'? Other components should be examined including: how it works, the outcomes, context, replication, appropriateness and acceptability.

Advantages of using the evidence base in practice can ensure that time, money, people and resources are directed effectively. Tang et al. (2003) propose that interventions often will find it difficult to obtain policy support if they do not have evidence of effectiveness. Tones and Green (2004) also argue that evidence can provide some back-up resistance and support for proposed policies or programmes that practitioners may not agree with.

WHAT EVIDENCE CAN BE USED?

The concept of evidence-based practice implies a rational, logical or sequential concept, starting with problem identification, moving to selection of intervention, then implementation (Harrison 2003). Rarely are the processes so simple. The first argument to disrupt this logical sequence is what evidence should be selected to start off this process?

It has been argued that only randomized control trials or systematic reviews should be used to inform the evidence base in health promotion, alongside the use of observational studies (Wang et al. 2005). Unfortunately, lack of resources mean that not all aspects of health can be tested in this way and it only gives a partial overview of the problem being identified, particularly when an intervention includes social or economic conditions. Literacy, acceptability, appropriateness, lack of resources, time and funding in addition to no trained staff can all impact on an intervention that attempts to be replicated in another area.

It is a challenge to health promotion to find evidence that is relevant to the topic area and avoids the reductionism notions that pervade the evidence base. The move to develop an evidence base through clinical practice has been heavily supported through government and medical organizations. Unfortunately this enthusiasm has not been replicated in health promotion. However, growing practical experience is increasing the notion of 'best practice' in health promotion and leading to more success (Nutbeam 1999).

The more traditional uses of evidence through clinical trials are not the only source that health promoters can use. Tang et al. (2003) propose four classifications of evidence that could be used in health promotion (Figure 7.2).

---

1   **Evidence that meets scientific fact criteria**, i.e. replicable, proven or repeatable over time.
2   **Evidence that has success and can be predicted**, but can only be replicated at local level in a certain time frame and only then if resources or certain settings are available.
3   **Evidence that has success but does not meet causality criteria**, but can be repeatable.
4   **Evidence that has success and can be predicted**, but does not meet causality criteria and can only be replicated at local level in a certain time frame and only then if resources or certain settings are available, and thus universal application is not achievable.

Figure 7.2   Four classifications of evidence used in health promotion, based on Tang et al. (2003)

Tang et al.'s (2003) classifications in Figure 7.2 illustrate four main classifications of evidence. This ranges from evidence that meets 'scientific' facts, to that which can be replicated under certain conditions, to evidence that is repeatable, but not controlled. Finally, evidence that is successful and can be predicted, providing it is applied to local levels if it meets certain criteria and conditions.

Activity 7.2:   What evidence do you use?

1   Using Figure 7.2 to help you in your health promotion work, which category of evidence do you use the most? Alternatively, if you are a student studying towards a health related programme, which evidence have you used the most for your assessments?

The NHS Centre for Reviews and Dissemination (2001) provides a similar hierarchy of research evidence that can also be used in health care practice. Wiggers and Sanson-Fisher (2001) place this into a number of levels.

Figure 7.3 illustrates the levels of evidence that could be included in health promotion. Clinical decision making tends to be based on level 1; at least one appropriately designed randomized control trial. However, health promotion frequently will find itself using levels 3 and 4; large comparable differences within time or location, and opinions of authority groups, descriptive studies or reports. This is often because the evidence simply does not exist at the higher levels (1 and 2), but also because health promotion fundamentally takes a holistic view of health and some health topics do not fit comfortably under the heading of a randomized control trial. Whatever figure we choose to favour, Figures 7.2 and 7.3 serve to illustrate that health promotion interprets a wider picture of health (not just the clinical trial-related one) and therefore most practitioners will use a combination of evidence from a number of levels.

Level 1:   At least one appropriately designed randomized control trial
Level 2a: Well-designed controlled trial without randomization
Level 2b: Well-designed cohort study
Level 2c: Well-designed case control study
Level 3:   Large comparable differences in time/location with/without the interventions
Level 4:   Opinions of authority groups with clinical experience, descriptive studies and reports

---

Figure 7.3   Levels of research evidence, based on Wiggers and Sanson-Fisher (2001)

Activity 7.3:   Planning with evidence

You are planning a community-based project in a small local neighbourhood to try to reduce theft and mugging in the area, which is unusually high. The residents identify poor street-lighting and nothing for 'youths' to do as the problem. The local council proposes community police officers as the solution. There are no randomized control trials or systematic reviews demonstrating the link between any of these solutions (street lights, 'bored' youths or community police officers) to the problem.

1   What do you think you would do to address the issue?
2   What evidence will you base this on?

Like other health interventions (for example, clinical practice), health promotion is made up of a linked ladder of activities, with national policies at the top, down to individual health promotion programmes at local level. The basic question of evidence-based practice – 'Does it work?' – may be posed at these different levels. Collecting evidence 'is the end result of processes for filtering, reviewing and synthesising research studies' (Marks 2003: 6), something that requires skill and practice. There are a number of sources available to the health practitioner to enable access in evidence-based practice.

THE YOUNG@HEART EVIDENCE-BASED INITIATIVE

A good example of evidence being used to influence national policies in a key area of health promotion can be found in the work of the National Heart Forum and its Young@heart initiative (Giles 2003). The National Heart Forum, a body made up of over 45 national organizations concerned with the prevention of coronary heart disease, commissioned an extensive review of the research on the early origins of coronary heart disease and the potential for reducing the risk and promoting health from early life and throughout childhood (Giles 2003). The initiative's 'Scientific and policy review' covered a wide range of clinical, genetic and socio-economic matters and likened these to the key issue of communicating effectively with children and young people. It also set this evidence in the context of an extensive body of existing government policies and initiatives, which impacted on the long-term coronary wellbeing of children and young people. Some of the topic areas surveyed in this collection and review of evidence are shown in Figure 7.4 as undertaken by a selection of experts in the field.

- The foetal and infant origins of coronary heart disease
- Socioeconomic position and coronary heart disease risk factors in children and young people
- Health-related behaviour in low-income families
- The diets of children and young people: implications for coronary heart disease prevention
- Determinants of young people's participation in physical activity
- Investigation of tracking of physical activity from youth to adulthood
- Policy implications for reducing smoking in young people
- Health promotion for young people in primary care: what works and what doesn't
- Children and young people: their social context and attitudes to smoking, physical activity and diet.

Figure 7.4   Example of topic areas surveyed in the Young@Heart review (Giles 2003)

The key concerns that emerged from the scientific review were:

- Poor diets among infants, children and young people.
- Lack of physical activity among children and young people.
- Persistent rates of smoking among teenagers.

The evidence-based approach to the Young@heart initiative enabled the National Heart Forum to develop its own policy framework, which has formed the basis of the Forum's policy advocacy work. The policy framework proposed a common health promoting agenda for departments across government and for agencies, partnerships and organizations working at both national and local levels across the public and commercial sectors. These included proposals for a national plan for children's and young people's health and wellbeing, with a particular focus on coronary heart disease prevention, and recommendations to develop comprehensive national strategies for improving nutrition, increasing physical activity, and tackling smoking among children and young people.

Clearly the scope and scale of the issue being addressed by the National Heart Forum and the level of resources available for the Young@Heart initiative go beyond the normal remit of individual health promotion practitioners and local programme developers. However, the key message from this work derives from its attempt to amass, evaluate and apply evidence relevant to the totality of the issue it was addressing. Hence the evidence sought related to four important areas of evidence-based practice:

- The clinical context.
- The socio-economic context.
- The government policy context.
- The robustness of the means of effective two-way communication with key stakeholders (in this case children and young people).

The same principles of research evidence informing policy and practice can be seen in operation in the development of local health promotion activities too. The Havering Primary Care Trust, under its 'Active Ageing' banner, operates a Healthy Lifestyles Club at locations in its area aimed at reducing and preventing falls among an at-risk group of referred clients (Havering PCT 2004). The programme was developed following research that shows the type of activity people need to do to stop themselves from falling.

WHERE TO FIND EVIDENCE?

Electronic bibliographic databases

Electronic bibliographic database use is on the increase by health practitioners via access to the Internet. Practitioners can make use of databases that have a focus on clinical, public health and health promotion issues such as the Cochrane Library, which published systematic reviews of information and the Campbell Collaboration, which contains evidence on randomized trials, interventions and evaluations.

Electronic or paper journals

Electronic or paper journals are another way of finding information for evidence-based practice. The *British Medical Journal* (*BMJ*) was one of the first databases to appear online with free access. There are a large number of national and international journals available in the areas of health promotion, health education and public health. For example, Oxford journals publish journals online including *Health Education Research*, *Health Policy and Planning* and *Health Promotion International*. Other journals include those that are designed to be accessed online. Bandolier is a free independent journal about evidence-based health care. Emerald Insight provide a free access range of journals online, some of which are useful for the health practitioner.

Government and other organization documentation

Governments in the developed world are usually well resourced to be able to access, collect and codify evidence in health and health care areas of activity. In the UK, the Health Development Agency (HDA) was established as a Special Health Authority in 2000, following the publication of *Saving lives: our healthier nation* (DOH 1999). The HDA's functions were transferred to the National Institute for Clinical Excellence in 2005, but the responsibilities and corresponding activities continue in broadly similar forms. Swann et al. (2005) describe the HDA's processes for the construction and dissemination of an evidence base across a wide and increasing range of health promotion areas. In fulfilment of one of the Agency's core functions, the building of an evidence base in public health and health improvement, particularly with regard to the effective reduction in health inequalities, the HDA developed a web-based database with a view to disseminating the best available evidence on what works to improve health and to reduce health inequalities.

Having developed its evidence briefing methodology, the HDA has published a series of 'Evidence briefings' covering a wide range of areas (see Figure 7.5). *The National Institute for Health and Clinical Excellence (NICE)* retains these ◀◀ evidence briefings as well as providing new reviews and the development of guidelines, interventions and technology appraisals of further health related topics (NICE 2006a).

- Accidental injury
- Alcohol misuse
- Drug use prevention
- Health impact assessment
- HIV prevention
- Obesity and overweight
- Physical activity
- Prevention of sexually transmitted infections
- Smoking and public health
- Suicide prevention

Figure 7.5   A list of examples of evidence briefings from the HDA (NICE 2006a)

Activity 7.4:　NICE evidence base

1　Visit www.nice.org.uk and select 'Guidance'. What documentation is available in the public health section that could be used to help design small- or large-scale health promotion campaigns?

Despite the emphasis on, and effort directed to, the collection of the best available evidence, there is also recognition within government that the best may be the enemy of the good. NICE, in an internal paper (NICE 2005), questioned the rigid application of hierarchies of evidence. It focussed on the question of whether it was more important to implement a recommendation based on high-quality evidence rather than one supported by a lower level of evidence, regardless of the effect, size or other factors that may determine its impact on health. As a result it was decided that NICE would no longer publish the classification grade of the evidence which supported its guidelines and recommendations. In effect NICE would be able to decouple its assessment of the quality of its evidence from the importance of its recommendations.

UK government publications also recognize that in some specific areas there may simply be no 'good' evidence to work with. In the NICE *evidence into practice briefing on promotion of physical activity* (Cavill et al. 2006), it is suggested that there are areas where it is not possible to suggest review level evidence-based actions or interventions, such as:

- physical activity intervention studies with people from black and ethnic minorities; and
- physical activity intervention reviews among people with physical limitations.

However, in both cases experienced practitioners in the respective fields were able to identify a number of themes of inquiry.

Grey literature

Grey literature refers to informal published material, which by its nature does not fit into a clearly identifiable group. This can include local reports such as those produced by NHS groups or Primary Care Trusts (PCTs) and conference proceedings. The use of local needs assessments, health impact assessments (HIA) or community profiles may help in identifying problems from a qualitative prospective. Networks may also be available where practitioners can share ideas.

Grey literature can be difficult to find and has been described as the proverbial needle in a haystack (Matthews 2004). However, useful material can often be found on the websites of relevant organizations and, increasingly, databases of grey literature are being established. An example of such a database is the Library of Grey Literature maintained by the West Midlands Public Health

Observatory, some of which is publicly available. Users of grey literature will need to satisfy themselves of the quality of documents accessed unless specific information is available on quality criteria checking.

Activity 7.5: Grey literature

1 What grey literature could you use in your work?
2 Have you compiled any materials that could be counted under the 'grey litera-ture' heading?

PROBLEMS WITH USING THE EVIDENCE BASE

Although there are many positive uses and justifications for evidence-based practice, there are also a number of problematic areas with the application of evidence, in particular to the discipline of health promotion. First, evidence alone cannot constitute good practice. Tang et al. (2003) argue that evidence can inform practice, but not produce practice. Without skilled practitioners who are able to find, locate and apply the evidence, interventions will be unable to fully utilize the evidence base.

Another issue is that the relevance of using the evidence base for a practitioner will depend on the quality of the evidence and how it can be implemented (Tones and Green 2004). Not all evidence is applicable to practice, in particular the use of some of the more traditionally proposed evidence bases (for example, randomised control trials). Traditional evidence and the theories or models of health that they are based on (in particular the biomedical model) may not be appropriate in the application to health promotion (Raphael 2000). Health promotion supposes a holistic definition of health and operates in a context of social, political and environmental influences, which more traditional evidence may have ignored. Evidence also is inclined to include a distinct Western bias to evidence, and material from a non-Western perspective is sparse (McQueen 2000, 2002). Application to groups who are non-Western therefore may be difficult or inappropriate.

Developing countries can be particularly problematic; some countries have less well-established evidence bases and may rely on other countries for evidence. Economic, social or political environments may be more complex in these areas, with less funding or resources available (Overseas Development Institute 2006). But does this imply that evidence based health promotion is simply a creation of the West, which has nothing to learn from the experiences of developing countries? McQueen (2000) reports the proceedings of an ad hoc group of attendees at the Fifth Conference on Global Health Promotion in Mexico City in 2000. He proposes that in the context of prolific debate on health promotion evidence in the Western world, there was a clear lack of participation from those representing the experience of the developing world. Underlying reasons for this exclusion were:

- the conduct of the debate in the English language by Europeans and Americans, or others educated there; and
- a restriction on participation in the debate largely to the academic elite or those privileged to hold the type of government offices that allow them involvement.

The ad hoc group thought that 'missing voices' should be uncovered and the evidence from developing nations brought into full play. To support this aim a set of recommendations was made (see Figure 7.6). These include establishing a working group, incorporating unpublished materials, consideration of alternative evaluation methods, alongside representation of a multi-cultural working group.

---

1 **The WHO should establish a workgroup** that will be responsible for creating a plan for the development of evaluation globally.
2 **This workgroup should build on work previously done** by other workgroups and integrate unpublished work into evaluation knowledge.
3 **Evaluation approaches should recognize the importance of equity** in conducting locally determined evaluation, and should emphasize the use of participatory approaches and multi-sectoral involvement in evaluation.
4 **The workgroup should have diverse cultural representation.**

Figure 7.6 Four recommendations to include developing nations in the development of an evidence base

---

Activity 7.6: Including developing countries

Read the four recommendations in Figure 7.6.

1 What problems can you foresee in following these recommendations?
2 How could these problems be overcome to include developing nations into evidence-based practice?

There have been some examples of the inaccurate use or misreporting of evidence. Cummins and Macintyre (2002) cite the example of 'food deserts' (see Case Study 7.1) where some ideas have been replicated as fact, even though they might not be true. They refer to these facts as 'factoids'; imagined or speculated facts that become true. Health practitioners are encouraged not just to assume evidence is true, but to question facts.

Case Study 7.1   Food deserts

Food deserts are areas where residents (in urban areas) do not have access to an affordable, healthy diet. Acheson (1998) in the *Independent inquiry into inequalities in health* hailed food deserts as an example of a way through which poverty could cause poor health in residents who lived in these areas. The Social Exclusion Unit (1998) supported this by postulating that food was often more expensive and less available in more deprived areas. These claims were based on studies, however, where results have been misinterpreted. The Acheson report did not include full findings that indicated food in deprived areas may not be more expensive. The SEU also did not provide any evidence to support strongly the finding that unhealthy food is less expensive than health food. They also did not cite any evidence that indicated food 'systematically' costs more in deprived areas (Cummins and Macintyre 2002). (See also Chapter 8 for food deserts.)

Some evidence can be very difficult to translate into practice, and McQueen (2002) suggests that lack of detail in relation to transferability can hinder the application of evidence-based practice to health promotion. Wang et al. (2005) also propose that it may be unethical to wait for evidence from actual local settings, for example in HIV. If there is a major public health issue (for example, infectious disease) that needs to be addressed quickly, the wait for evidence can be lengthy.

ACCEPTABILITY AND TRANSFERABILITY

Implementation is an important part of using evidence-based practice (Newman and Harrier 2006). Health promotion practice sometimes has difficulties translating the evidence base into a practical programme, so even if the evidence exists replication may be unclear. There is little point of a study advocating good practice if a practitioner cannot then replicate this. Evidence-based practice should be able to be replicated in a different place and a different time (Harrison 2003). One of the problems with this is that interventions are often population- or location-specific and are difficult to replicate in a different context. Transferring evidence to 'local circumstance, local capacity, local ownership and local obstacles to implementation' (Marks 2003: 23) is a challenge for health practitioners.

There has been some interest in the problems associated with applicability of evidence in evidence-based practice, alongside some of the factors associated at local levels that impact on transferability (Sharp 2005). One proposal to take advantage of the wealth of evidence based information is to apply a criterion to see if the intervention is acceptable and transferable to current practice.

	Applicability
1	Does the political environment allow this intervention? Are there any political barriers to implementation?
2	Would the population accept this intervention? Does the intervention go against any social norms or ethical principles?
3	Can the contents be tailored for the intervention group?
4	Are there resources to implement this intervention?
5	Does the target group have sufficient educational levels to understand the intervention?
6	Which organization will provide this intervention? Are there barriers in this organization to implementing this intervention?
7	Do the providers have the skills to deliver the intervention?
	Transferability
8	What is the base-line prevalence of the health problem? What is the difference between the study setting and the target setting?
9	Are the characteristics similar between the study and the target population? Will demographics such as age, socioeconomic status etc. impact on the effectiveness of the intervention?
10	Is the capacity to implement the intervention comparable between the study and the target area in political enviroment, acceptability, resources, delivery structure and skills of providers?

Figure 7.7   Questions to ask in determining applicability and tranferability, based on Wang et al. (2005) © Oxford University Press

Wang et al. (2005) propose a practical approach to getting evidence based findings into practice in different contexts via a series of acceptability and transferability questions.

Each question covers key areas that may make the difference between success and failure in health promotion practice. Figure 7.7 allows the selection of a study, where the practitioner can then ask a series of questions to see if that study can successfully be replicated in practice. This does not guarantee instant success as wider variables may mitigate circumstances, but it does go some way to covering the pitfalls associated with the replication of other's work. Wang et al. (2005) propose that after the questions in Figure 7.7 have been applied, there are likely to be four outcomes. First, that the intervention finds little difference between the study setting and the target setting and the intervention will demonstrate health outcomes should it be implemented. Second, the intervention could meet the requirements with additional work, for example, some minor adjustments to the original study. Third, there may not be enough evidence to apply transferability or applicability information, and more research is required. Last, there may be a considerable difference between the study group and the target group, and the application of the study is inappropriate. Another approach should be adopted in this instance, either by working towards implementation of the study at a later date or by choosing another approach to the problem.

Case Study 7.2   Acceptability and transferability design

'Bones in mind' was an osteoporosis programme run by the Woman's Institute (WI) with Cornwall and the Isles of Scilly Health Promotion Department in a predominately white, rural area in 1999. This programme trained a number of older women from the WI to deliver a 10-week programme. The 10-week programme was attended by members of the local WI in the local area. The women in the groups ranged between 40–70 years. The WI provided the local halls and refreshments for the sessions. Training, publicity materials and other costs were paid for by the local health promotion department. The sessions ran once a week for 2 hours and included weight-bearing physical activity regimens, nutritional activities and advice. Informal evaluation indicated that women were more likely to eat calcium-rich foods and partake in physical activity at follow-up, compared to when they first joined the programme.

(Cornwall and IOS Health Authority 1999)

Activity 7.7:   Acceptability and transferability

You are working for a local health promotion organization. Your target group is: Women 30–50, in an inner-city area, predominately Asian and white, some of whom are non-English speaking. There are some local women's groups who have expressed an interest in an osteoporosis programme, but your health promotion department has no additional funding to help you. You do have access to a physical activity coordinator who usually works with children and who is willing to help you.
Look again at the 'Applicability and transferability questions' in Figure 7.7.

1   Can you apply the Cornwall and the Isles of Scilly 'Bones in mind' (Case Study 7.2) osteoporosis programme to the new target group?
2   Is there anything you might need to do to make sure the programme is successful?

HOW TO ESTABLISH AN EVIDENCE BASE

One of the problems with application of an evidence-based approach is the lack of evidence available. Harrison (2003) argues that this difficultly arises because different disciplines and practices contribute different approaches, analysis or collection to the evidence base. One of the roles of a health practitioner is therefore not just to utilize the existing evidence base, but to apply consistent methods to practice, and to add other evidence through practice to inform future health promotion work.

Nutbeam (1999) highlights four ways that best practice can be achieved (see Figure 7.8) and thus lead to providing evidence of effectiveness. He suggests that if these processes are in place, there will be greater success of objectives and thus the intervention. Alongside this there will be a greater likelihood that the intervention will be able to be added to the existing evidence base, and thus inform future practice.

1	**Analyse** epidemiological, behavioural and social research in planning the intervention
2	**Use established theories** that are appropriate to the intervention planned to develop the programme
3	**Ensure that conditions are favourable** for the intervention, including resources, training, services, capacity etc.
4	**Implement the intervention in a sample** of suitable size and sufficient duration to enable results to be identified over other variables.

Figure 7.8   Four ways that best practice can be achieved, adapted from Nutbeam (1999)

According to Figure 7.8, the first way best practice can be achieved is through the analysis of epidemiological, social or other research to assist in the planning of the intervention. This means using evidence-based policy and practice – as Harrison (2003) suggested earlier – to make a judgement or decision on the most appropriate intervention(s). The second way of ensuring best practice is to use established theories (Chapter 1 provides a detailed account of ways to use these theories). The third way is to ensure favourable conditions. Supportive environments and conducive conditions, as well as well-stocked resources, are more likely to herald success. Last, the intervention should be implemented over a large enough intervention and for long enough duration to enable results to be demonstrated that can be attributed to the project and not to other variables, for example, another project. By following designs for best practice, the likelihood of a successful intervention that can be replicated by others is higher.

USING AN EVIDENCE BASE TO IDENTIFY METHODS AND STRATEGIES

'Turning evidence into practice depends on the quality of evidence, its accessibility, effective methods for dissemination, and a context which favours implementation of effective interventions' (Marks 2003: 4). Evidence that is available for health practitioners covers a wide range of areas, and a health practitioner working in the areas covered should be aware of the evidence base for their particular line of work. The reviews themselves can cover good practice, methods that work best in target groups, strategies to reduce certain aspects of health-related problems and other key evidence for successful health promotion work.

Newman and Harrier (2006) propose that one of the most important things a practitioner must do in using the evidence is to ask questions. They provide a list of ways evidence could be used, based on research by Sackett et al. (1996). Some of these questions are applicable to health promotion practice. These include using evidence to identify:

- causes of problems;
- goals or aims of interventions;
- ways to reduce occurrences of ill health;
- ways to improve health; and
- perceptions of others (for example, the target group).

Sometimes causes of problems need to be identified to be able to highlight issues to focus on. For example, perhaps young people smoke because they want to impress their peers, or think it makes them look 'cool'. If this, or other reasons for smoking, can be identified, interventions can focus on the 'causes'. Formulation of goals, aims or objectives can be taken from evidence-based research. Evidence-based practice should be able to provide some suggestions of ways to overcome ill-health or improve health which can be adapted for practice. And finally, evidence can give practitioners perceptions and ideas about the proposed target group that can support their own work with the target group.

One of the most straightforward ways to identify appropriate interventions or target groups from evidence is to utilize recommendations from national organizations. The NICE Internet database contains a large number of recommendations and guidance, as highlighted earlier. In the area of smoking cessation, NICE has made a number of recommendations for stop-smoking practice. These include the recommendations listed in Figure 7.9 (NICE 2006b). Health practitioners, policy-makers and other health professionals are encouraged to put into action these recommendations. As a health promoter, this may mean selecting one or a combination of these recommendations for practice.

- Everyone who smokes should be advised to quit
- If an individual presents to a health service with a smoking related disease, advice could be linked to their condition
- Advice to stop smoking should be sensitive and tailored to individuals
- Those health care professionals who see smokers should offer referral to an intensive support service (i.e. stop smoking services)
- Smoking cessation advice and support should be available in the community, primary and secondary care settings
- Hard to reach groups should be targeted, alongside ethnic minority groups

---

Figure 7.9   A selection of evidence from NICE (2006b) for smoking cessation

---

Activity 7.8:   Evidence and smoking cessation

▶▶

Read the recommendations from the NICE (2006b) database for *'brief interventions
and referral for smoking cessation in primary care and other settings'* in Figure 7.9.
    You are a health promoter working in the area of smoking cessation and have a
small amount of money to spend on a stop-smoking project.

1   Based on the evidence, identify a target group, setting and appropriate inter-
    vention that you could undertake.

Practitioners should critically appraise health promotion literature to enable
interventions to be informed by the evidence base. Wiggers and Sanson-
Fisher (2001) propose that practitioners should examine literature critically to
determine four things: reliability, validity, acceptability and sensitivity. Thus
practitioners can ask questions of the research under these four headings.

Rada et al. (1999) propose that intervention information in health promotion
comes from two main sources: the target population and research based on other
populations. To ensure that health promotion interventions are successful, the
information required should come from both sources. To gain information about
the target population it is probable that sources may include: local morbidity or
mortality statistics, community profiles, needs assessments, interviews/focus
groups or other forms of local information. Undertaking these processes can be
represented as a circular model that a practitioner can move through before
achieving the final result (see Figure 7.10).

The basic steps in Figure 7.10 demonstrate the stages a practitioner could
move through to incorporate evidence-based practice into health promotion
work. An alternative linear model has been proposed by Levandowski et al.
(2006) based on a parental literacy program. These are simplistic steps, but they
give an idea of at what stage evidence is used in the planning and evaluation
processes. This model illustrates the fact that evidence is reviewed and analysed
throughout the intervention process. When the intervention is complete it is
evaluated, and these findings (either successful or unsuccessful) are then fed
back into the evidence base for the next health promotion project.

CONCLUSION

Health promotion should be in a position to promote and enable access to the
evidence base, particularly when IT allows wider access to materials. Marks
(2003) argues that 'the key to evidence-based practice … is that the evidence

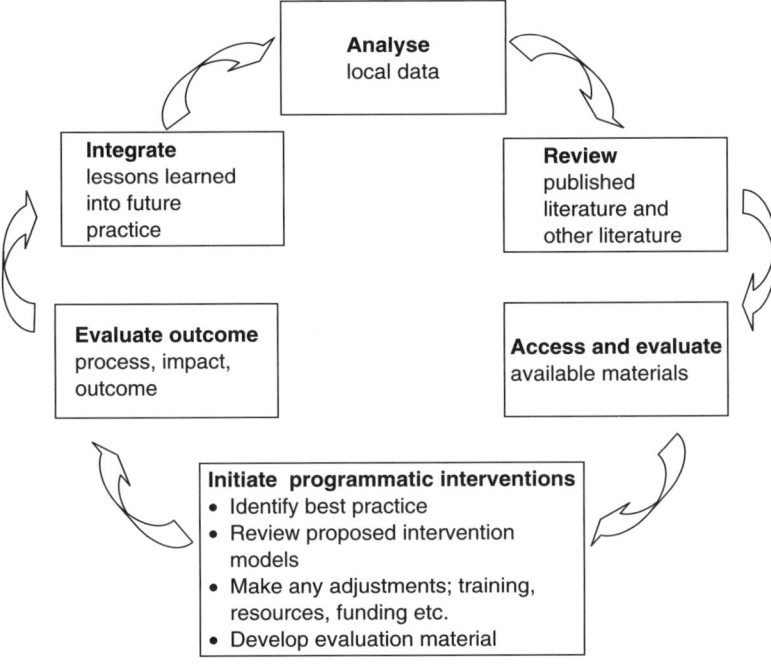

Figure 7.10   The steps for the inclusion of evidence-based practice, based on Levandowski et al. (2006)

base and review of effectiveness of interventions should be accessible and useful to decision makers' (Marks 2003: 28). This includes practitioners in non-Western countries who have been excluded or overlooked previously. Those who need evidence should be able to access what they need to make informed choices and decisions, and evidence should be made more accessible to those who need it and which have characteristics that enable interventions to be implemented (Sharp 2005).

The debate about the use (or non-use) of evidence-based practice should be taking a back seat to more productive discussions around the well-trodden grounds of the problems of using evidence. If practitioners want skills to implement and access evidence, why can they not be gained? (After all, the job of most health promoters is, to some extent, to give skills and knowledge to others). If evidence is not readily available – why is it not available? How can it be made more easily available? Other essential topics should include ways to move forward strategies to compile, use, apply, transfer and implement evidence-based practice into health promotion planning and programmes. Only when we see action will we start to see change.

Summary

- This chapter has highlighted the role of evidence-based practice in health promotion practice.
- The debates and issues surrounding the use of evidence and the current debates surrounding evidence-based practice have been highlighted.
- An applicability and transferability framework have been explored and applied to practice.
- Ways to establish and utilize evidence-based practice, including accessing evidence for practice and building up the evidence base in health promotion have been examined.

ADDITIONAL READING

An overview of evidence-based practice in health care is available from Gray, J A M (2001) *Evidence-based health* care, 2nd edition. Churchill Livingstone, London.

A broad textbook linking theory and research to evidence-based practice is Naidoo, J and Wills, J (2004) *Public health and health promotion: developing practice*: Bailliere Tindall, London.

The National Institute for Health and Clinical Excellence provides guidelines for practitioners including evidenced-based briefings and public health guidance in the UK. This is available at www.public health.nice.org.uk.

Using evaluation in health promotion communication

Sue Corcoran

Learning objectives:

- Explore models of evaluation theory in relation to communication processes in health promotion programmes.
- Apply theoretical models of evaluation to the practice setting.
- Identify strategies that would be required to plan an effective evaluation of communication within a health promotion programme or campaign.

It is important 'to know what we know what we know, and to know that we do not know what we do not know, that is true knowledge' (Nicholas Copernicus)

Evaluation can be defined simply as determining the value or assessing the worth of something. It has an increasingly important role in health promotion and is central to the development of a robust evidence base. Evaluating communication in health promotion can be complex and challenging, and it requires the practitioner to have available a toolbox of methods that will enable them to select a range of options that can be tailored to suit a particular activity. The bedrock of health promotion evaluation is the model of process, impact and outcome evaluation. This chapter explores evaluation in relation to communication processes within health promotion programmes and campaigns with an emphasis on the need for a multi-dimensional approach. It also considers methods to employ when presenting evaluation outcomes to stakeholders. Examples of good practice are given as well as opportunities for the application of the theoretical knowledge base.

DEFINING EVALUATION

Evaluation involves 'the determination of how successful a programme, a curriculum, a series of experiments, a drug, etc has been in achieving the goals laid out for it at the outset' (Reber 1985: 253). It often involves a range of methods that assist in gaining a more rounded view of the activity. The evaluation can be quantitative and/or qualitative, formal and informal. Evaluation of health promotion programmes tend to encompass all of these. At one level it may be incorporated into a practitioner's day-to-day activity in the form of appraisal and assessment, at another it is systematic, rigorous and formal and may be undertaken by outside researchers. Naidoo and Wills (2000) argue that evaluation is not a technical strategy but is a complex means of intervention which opens up debate with stakeholders measuring relationship with outcome.

Health promotion as a discipline is concerned with empowering individuals to take control and influence their own health. Providing evidence through evaluation requires the use of methods that reflect health promotion goals. These include equal access to health, involvement of stakeholders and the development of healthy public policy (Wright 1999). Evaluation of health promotion programmes is an important activity so that the body of evidence can be developed and disseminated. Plianbangchang, in his keynote address to the WHO Sixth Global Conference on Health Promotion, stated that 'establishment of a structured mechanism for policy and programme planning, monitoring and evaluation as well as documentation and dissemination of information shall be an integral part of all health promotion efforts at country and regional levels' (2005: 10). Previous chapters have discussed the challenges in defining the concept of health and its varying dimensions, thus health is defined within the context of individual, societal and environmental states. It is therefore unsurprising that any meaningful evaluation of health promotion will reflect a multifaceted approach.

There are a wealth of reasons why health promotion should be evaluated, as described in Figure 8.1, which illustrates that reasons for evaluation can fall under four categories: fiscal, quality, evidence and policy. 'Fiscal' reasons for evaluation include cost-effectiveness or legitimizing budgets. 'Quality' reasons could be ensuring accountability or effectiveness using performance indicators. 'Evidence' reasons for evaluation can be to increase the evidence base or improve what already works. 'Policy' reasons for evaluation include informing future planning or legitimizing decisions.

Health promotion evaluation often relates directly to the allocation and effective use of resources and seeks to legitimize policy decisions. Evaluation should also seek to improve the evidence base and understand the potential and limiting factors for success to enable improvement in future health promotion practice.

Type of evaluation	Example of evaluation
Fiscal	Cost effectiveness Allocation of resources Securing funding Legitimizing budget reduction
Quality	Assessing effectiveness using performance indicators Clinical governance to inform practice Recognizing the ethical dimensions of promoting health Ensuring accountability
Evidence	Increasing evidence base Developing theoretical concepts Improving methodologies Sharing experiences and understanding limitations
Policy	Informing future planning Legitimizing policy decisions Using for political ends Assisting in long-term strategies

Figure 8.1   Sixteen reasons for evaluating health promotion programmes, adapted from Katz et al. (2000) after Downie et al. (1992)

Activity 8.1:   Who is interested in evaluation?

You are planning to evaluate a campaign to provide facilities for mothers to breast-feed in shops and restaurants in a local town. Use the headings in Figure 8.1:

1   Which headings might be appropriate to an evaluation of this campaign?
2   Make a list of the people and organizations who would be most interested in the outcomes of the campaign.

WHY EVALUATE COMMUNICATION IN HEALTH PROMOTION?

All health promotion occurs within the context of communication. When looking at areas such as changes in behaviours, communication is a key component for achieving a successful outcome. Communication evaluation is an area that has received less attention, even though social psychological theory is acknowledged as being central to health promotion practice and assists in devising strategies (Bennett and Murphy 1997). Health communication, however, is being increasingly recognized as a discipline, using communication strategies to inform and influence individual and community decisions that enhance both personal and public health (Jackson and Duffy 1998).

The Ottawa Charter (WHO 1986) emphasized the importance of the involvement of people, families and communities in promoting and evaluating health. Lowell and Ziglio (2003) put forward the view that the principles of the charter must be reframed for application in the 21st century. They describe the importance of involving new partners in health promotion while acknowledging that huge inequalities in the relationship of the partners make it difficult to adopt notions of empowerment, equity, participation and ultimately health. Health promotion must create a collaborative or adaptive communication. In the light of this challenge we need to develop new models and frameworks of evaluation that will reflect the way that we communicate with all partners involved in shaping health policy and action.

Opportunities for using different approaches to the delivery of health education communication, particularly in areas such as the interactive media, has meant that it has become increasingly important to develop a reliable evidence base. It is argued that given the critical role that communication plays in all aspects of public health and health care, evaluation of health communication should be integrated across all health domains (US Office of Disease Prevention and Health Promotion 2000).

OVERVIEW OF MODELS AND THEORIES OF EVALUATION IN HEALTH PROMOTION

This section will consider a selection of theoretical models and theories for evaluation in health promotion that have been most commonly used for health promotion campaigns and programme evaluation. These include the process, impact and outcome model. This is the most commonly used evaluation method in health promotion; however, there are a number of other models that can be of use by the health practitioner in evaluating programmes. These include economic, pluralistic, participatory, experimental and social marketing evaluation.

PROCESS, IMPACT AND OUTCOME EVALUATION

Evaluation in health normally involves the bringing together of a variety of assessments, which help to define whether an activity has achieved its aims in the short- and longer-term and helps to describe how the aims were achieved. Evaluation should also be continued throughout the life of a programme and beyond to ensure that all elements of the programme are tested. The model of evaluation commonly used is that of process, impact and outcome evaluation illustrated in Figure 8.2.

Process evaluation is concerned with the journey taken by the programme. It focuses on all aspects of an intervention. It helps to describe and understand the implementation, and contributes towards the development of further learning and improved performance. It can assist in assessing the degree of success or failure of a programme (Platt et al. 2004). Process evaluation utilizes a wealth of methods that are both qualitative and quantitative and which often require direct contact with the individual or the community.

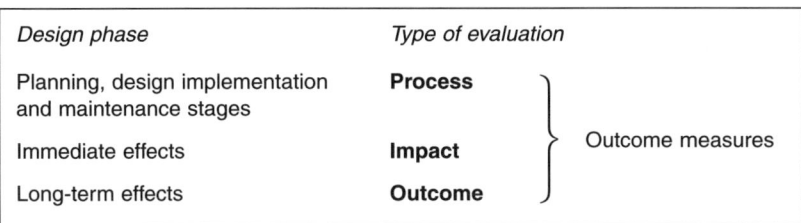

Figure 8.2 Process, impact and outcome evaluation

Impact evaluation has to answer the question 'Did it work?' It seeks to track actual change of status within a predetermined timeframe. It generally gives the stakeholders a signal that the programme is having an impact in the short term. It can be significant when determining issues such as whether knowledge and skills have been achieved or professional practice has changed as a result of the intervention. It may also provide the evidence that will support continuation of funding for a programme.

Outcome evaluation describes the effects of a programme over a longer period of time. Knowledge and skills of individuals can be measured by impact evaluation, but in outcome evaluation the application of these follows a continuum influenced by changes in health behaviours and expectations of health within a framework of environmental and socio-economic factors. The effects are usually measured by indicators such as quality of life, disability, morbidity and mortality and equity of access to services. Any evidence, for instance in reduction of morbidity or mortality, may not be seen for years (Nutbeam 1998). In summary, as proposed by Hawe et al. (1990):

- Programme goal is measured by *outcome evaluation.*
- Programme objective is measured by *impact evaluation.*
- Health promotion interventions and capacity building strategies are measured by *process evaluation.*

Case Study 8.1 Evaluation of a healthy village project in Malaysia

A project described by Kiyu et al. (2006) in 2000 was based on the WHO Healthy Village campaign. The project aimed to enable a population of ethnic minority groups who live in remote rural areas to improve their quality of life. The problems identified were poverty, a high incidence of communicable and non-communicable disease, accidents, injuries and environmental hazards.

(Continued)

The project analysis can be split into process, impact and outcome evaluation (this is not a definitive list):

Process evaluation
Participation
Implementation

Impact evaluation
Change in smoking habits
Change in exercise habits
Measurement of food hygiene

Outcome evaluation (indicated in the longer term)
Environmental improvements
Quality of life improvements
Reduction in morbidity and mortality

Activity 8.2:   Using process, impact and outcome evaluation

A programme has been set up to encourage people over the age of 50 to take more exercise in the form of walking.

1   Using the model of process impact and outcome evaluation, make a list of the ways you could demonstrate successful outcomes.

ECONOMIC EVALUATION

Economics in its simplest definition seeks to judge the allocation of scarce resources. In health promotion it is concerned with estimating the relative value of a programme or intervention in relation to its health benefit. Economic evaluation aims to assist policy-makers to set priorities, in the longer-term to improve efficiency by converting 'inputs' such as money or labour into 'outputs' such as health gain or saving lives. Economic evaluation uses a variety of tools such as cost-effective analysis, cost-benefit analysis and cost-utility analysis (see Figure 8.3). Cost-effective analysis proposes to measure consequences of interventions such as years gained or lives saved. Rationing or prioritizing would dictate how much the intervention is implemented. Cost-benefit analysis uses monetary terms and is centred around how much money is spent or saved; this is a broad form of evaluation. Lastly, cost-utility analysis is interested in both quality and quantity, the concept of adding years to life and life to years, rather

Type of analysis	Analysis philosophy
Cost effectiveness analysis	• Measures the consequences of health interventions in terms of natural or physical units, for example years of life gained • Does not question should we do the intervention but how much should we do
Cost benefit analysis	• Values consequences in monetary terms, for example how much have we saved? • Asks do the benefits outweigh the costs • Broadest form of economic evaluation
Cost utility analysis	• States of health are valued in relation to one another • Measure both quality and quantity of life

Figure 8.3   Cost-effectiveness, cost-benefit and cost-utility analysis, adapted from Miller (2001) with permission from Trent RDSU

than just quantitative measures. When evaluating health promotion interventions it is important to consider all three of these components.

PLURALISTIC EVALUATION

Pluralism can be defined as 'a situation within a state or social organization in which power is shared (or held to be shared) among a multiplicity of groups and organizations' (Jary and Jary 1991: 473). Pluralistic evaluation recognizes that when assessing the efficacy of an intervention each individual or group involved in the intervention will have a different perspective. All health promotion programmes will have a number of stakeholders whose influence and power on the outcomes of the programme will be unequal. Pluralistic evaluation seeks to challenge the idea that everyone wants the same things and there is a common set of values for the programme. By using a variety of methods and levels of involvement with all stakeholders in the planning implementation and evaluation, the programme will provide a rich source of evidence.

There is some scepticism expressed that sometimes lip service is paid to pluralistic evaluation due to different views on what information is important to capture. Israel and Chui (2006), when looking at interventions to improve health outcomes of prisoners, state that commitment to pluralistic evaluation in principle is often compromised in practice. The outcomes for health interventions for prisoners were measured by quantitative methods, for example, re-offending rates. The wider health benefits were not explored, such as the acceptability of the programme or changes in beliefs and values and Israel and Chui (2006) criticize this 'evaluation-driven practice'.

PARTICIPATORY EVALUATION

Participatory evaluation is the primary feature of community health-based programmes. It takes a pluralistic approach with the aim of ensuring that individuals within the community are not only benefiting from the programme but also participating in its planning implementation and evaluation. Participatory evaluation gives the opportunity to enable less articulate or disadvantaged individuals and groups to have an opportunity to influence the programme and its outcomes (Jones et al. 2002).

Case Study 8.2   Participatory evaluation in a neighbourhood

Primary school children were asked what they thought about their neighbourhood. Group and individual discussion was used as well as written work. It was then decided to give each child a disposable camera.
    They were asked to photograph:

- Their favourite place.
- The places they avoided.
- The places that were part of their families' daily lives.

The photographs were displayed locally, using the children's own words to describe them (Green 1994).

Activity 8.3:   Participatory evaluation in action

A group of primary school children are participating in a healthy eating programme. This includes a project where the children are learning to grow vegetables in the school allotment. Two of the aims of the programme for the children are:

- To understand how vegetables are grown.
- To understand the health benefits of eating vegetables.

What participatory evaluation methods could you use to demonstrate achievement of these aims?

SOCIAL MARKETING

Social marketing is often used to enhance the effect of mass communication. It is defined as 'the use of marketing principles and techniques to influence a target audience to voluntarily accept, reject, modify or abandon a behaviour for the benefit of individuals, groups or society as a whole' (Kotler et al. 2002: 5) (Chapter 4 covers social marketing in more depth). It is argued that if marketing can persuade people to buy fast foods, clothing or other products worldwide, then a similar approach within health promotion could persuade individuals and groups to adopt healthier behaviours. Social marketing can influence behaviours of not just individuals but of policy-makers, governments and influential interest groups (Macfayden et al. 1999). The wide influence of social marketing can be illustrated by evaluation of large health campaigns in developing countries where mass communication is widely used. Case Study 8.3 is an example of this in action.

Case Study 8.3   Social marketing and UNICEF

The UNICEF Water and Environmental Sanitation (WES) project in India 1966–1998 sent drilling equipment for wells to drought-ridden areas of India. The project later expanded to include sanitation and hygiene awareness.

During the evaluation of the WES projects it was recognized that women played a vital role in promoting the health of their villages and for a large part of the day were involved in carrying water, food preparation and childcare responsibilities. They also found that sometimes discrimination and traditional practices undermined women's health and wellbeing.

One of the recommendations from the projects was to introduce gender-specific training into programmes in order to encourage UNICEF workers to understand the roles and perceptions of men and women within their particular societal norms. Through the evaluation a framework was developed to compile the questions that needed to be addressed when implementing future programmes. These included:

- Have training programmes given women the opportunity to examine their position in society, the burden of water carrying on their lives, and the effect on their daughters' schooling?
- Is the community aware of the unequal burden?
- Have men gained a greater sense of sharing responsibilities?
- Can women maintain water systems?
- Are women involved in the planning and implementation of projects?

UNICEF propose that in future projects the role of social marketing will be used to enhance the success of their future programmes.

(UNICEF 2000)

EXPERIMENTAL DESIGN EVALUATION

Experimental evaluation in health generally compares the success of an intervention by making comparisons with those who have been exposed to an intervention to those who have not. It also can measure the before-and-after effects of a programme and tends to report on specific health outcomes. The application of this type of evaluation involves establishing 'variables', which can be defined as characteristics, such as age or gender, that may influence any result. Randomized controlled trials (RCTs) are seen as the most reliable method of experimental evaluation in health. There are two main tenets of an RCT: people are randomly allocated to a study group, and there needs to be at least two groups for comparison. They are widely used in therapeutic decision making, for example, clinical trials for determining the efficacy of a drug regime. RCTs are generally considered to be unable to cope with the complexity of health promotion programmes; for example, they cannot measure process outcomes and are incompatible with active individual and community participation (Tones and Green 2004). Health promotion evaluation methods are required, however, to compete with these so-called scientific methods to gain credibility as a discipline (Thorogood and Coombes 2004).

An example of this is 'Heartbeat Wales', which attempted to set up a 'control' group of participants in a region of England to act as a comparator to the Welsh experimental group. They acknowledged that they could not prevent contact between the two groups and assumed any contact might just dilute the findings. In fact, it resulted in compromising the impacts of the study (Nutbeam 1993). In today's society, our access in communication channels such as telephone and Internet and our social mobility can mitigate against comparing population outcomes in health promotion interventions.

Reliability and validity

Effectiveness of research outcomes are usually measured in terms of their reliability. Reliability is concerned with achieving consistent results even when the activity is repeated. For example, observation of behaviours of a group of teenagers when confronted with a poster about chlamydia infection would not alter if viewed by a second observer. Another aspect of ensuring that findings are credible is through the use of internal and external validity measurement. Internal validity measures the extent to which the results are deemed accurate due to the intervention itself and not other factors; in other words, the right things were measured. External validity is concerned with how the results can be extrapolated for a wider use. If, for example, a programme to improve the dental hygiene practices of a group of 5-year-olds in a school in Birmingham resulted in a 50 per cent improvement in their tooth-brushing technique, can it be assumed that similar results would be achieved if the programme was repeated in a school in Manchester?

Activity 8.4: Validity in evaluation

A group of men between the ages of 50 and 60 are recruited onto a weight-reduction programme. One group embarks on a healthy eating programme while a second group undertakes an exercise programme.

1 Make a list of the problems you may encounter when assessing internal and external validity in your evaluation of this programme.
2 What strategies could improve validity?

It has already been acknowledged that evaluation in health promotion needs to reflect the complexity of how people communicate within health promotion programmes. It has also been demonstrated that some models of evaluation may work better than others. Complexity, however, should not detract from the achievement of sound, high-quality evaluation. Cummings and Macintyre (2002) criticize the over-interpretation of small-scale studies in health promotion. They postulate that health policy is sometimes determined by 'factoids', which are assumptions or speculations repeated over time that end up being assumed to be true in the absence of empirical evidence. They cite the so-called 'food deserts' in poor urban areas, which are assumed to exist and which are perceived to be a major reason for poor nutrition among the socially disadvantaged (more information on 'factoids' can be found in Chapter 7).

EVALUATING INTERVENTIONS USING THEORETICAL MODELS OF COMMUNICATION

Chapter 1 explored theoretical models of communication and their application to health promotion practice. In this section, examples are used that demonstrate how these models can be used to evaluate health communication. Theoretical models help to frame the planning and evaluation process. In practice, however, they are often modified or used in conjunction with each other. This helps to avoid the pitfalls of applying a rigid framework to a complex area of predicting human behaviour and experience. Theoretical models also help to take into account the variables that will influence programme outcomes (Tones and Green 2004). In an Australian study of how helpful theoretical models were to health promotion practitioners, it appeared that they found models to be more use in the early conceptual phase of planning than in the 'action' phases of implementation and evaluation (Jones and Donovan 2004).

Papadaki and Scott (2006) report on an evaluation of a healthy eating website. Using the process model of evaluation, they used elements of the health belief model and theory of planned behaviour (see Chapter 1) to assist in developing the website. They considered barriers, self-efficacy skills, attitudes and social influences in the design. The website was evaluated over a six-month period using a triangulation approach, allowing data to be cross-referenced to provide a more objective measure of outcomes. In this study they included website visit numbers, questionnaires and focus group interviews. The results demonstrated that the website was viewed as being interesting, informative, novel, trustworthy, easy to understand, useful, user-friendly, attractive and encouraging.

A study in Tanzania (Vaughan and Rogers 2000) used a variety of models to create a staged model through which communication messages have effects on individual behaviour change. They drew on various theories including the stages of change model (or the transtheoretical model; see Chapter 1) and diffusion of innovations theory. They looked at involvement with media characters and role-modelling of their actions and at interpersonal communication. Data from the field experiment on the effects of an educational radio soap opera 'Twende na Wakati' ('Let's go with the times') on the take-up of family planning are analysed in the light of a six stage model of communication effects. They found that the model was useful in providing a framework for understanding the effects of this type of education programme and found that the radio soap opera improved the take-up of family planning methods during three of the four years of broadcast, and this outcome was replicated when the soap opera was broadcast in another area of Tanzania.

Diffusion innovation theory (Rogers 1983) is used as a way of describing new ideas and what effect they have on behaviours. It acknowledges that messages are interpreted and exchanged through social networks. It is suggested that the behaviour change can be achieved by a 'top-down' approach where innovations are developed and filtered down. There is evidence to show that health coalition groups such as the Terence Higgins Trust and ASH are also as effective (Murphy and Bennett 2002). Peer health education is an example of the application of diffusion innovation theory. Initiatives with young people are used widely, as the educators are seen to share the beliefs and values of the client group. It is argued, however, that the peer educators are presenting an 'adult' view imposed on a captive audience (Milburn 1995). (Chapter 1 covers theoretical models in more depth, and Chapter 2 examines messages and young people in more detail.)

Case Study 8.4   Peer education and HIV

A peer education in HIV prevention project in schools in Athens, Greece, was implemented (Merakou and Kourea-Kremastinou 2006). A survey aimed to test the effectiveness of peer education methods in HIV prevention. 702 students from 13 schools were divided into an intervention group and a control group. Peer education was given to the intervention group and both groups were tested using anonymous questionnaires. Compared with the control group, the intervention group were slightly more empowered to:

- increase their personal responsibility; and
- adopt safer behaviours in sexual practice.

There was no significant change in knowledge, in attitude to condom use, initiation of sexual relations or discrimination about particular groups of people between groups. The conclusions were that peer education can influence personal behaviour with regard to protection from HIV infection, but that peer education needs further evaluation as to its effectiveness for behavioural change.

WHAT TO MEASURE

One of the key questions that health promotion practitioners have to ask is what should actually be measured when evaluating effective health communication? *Healthy people 2010* (US Office of Disease Prevention and Health Promotion 2000) suggest a number of key elements in assessing whether health communication has been effective. Figure 8.4 illustrates these. Key elements cover accuracy, availability, balance, consistency, cultural competence, evidence base,

Accuracy	Is the content valid? Are there any errors of fact?
Availability	Is the content delivery or placement accessible?
Balance	Does the content present the benefits and risks (or both sides of the issue)?
Consistency	Is the content consistent over time?
Cultural competence	Does the whole design process account for variables such as ethnicity, race and language?
Evidence base	Has the relevant evidence undergone analysis and review to formulate practice guidelines?
Reach	Does the information reach the whole target population?
Reliability	Are sources of content credible and up to date?
Repetition	Is delivery or access to information continued or repeated to reinforce impact?
Timeliness	Is content available or provided when the audience is most in need of it or most receptive to it?
Understandability	Is the reading language or format appropriate?

Figure 8.4 Suggestions for the evaluation of effective health communication, adapted from *Healthy People 2010* (US Office of Disease Prevention and Health Promotion 2000)

reach, reliability, repetition, timeliness and understandability. It is easy to see how questions could be fitting around these elements. For example, if you wanted to measure accuracy, you could ask if the content is correct and whether it contains validated facts. If you wanted to measure reach, you could question if the content reaches everyone for whom the information is intended.

Activity 8.5:   Ways to evaluate health communication

1   Using the headings in Figure 8.4, how you would plan to evaluate a campaign to promote use of newly opened cycle lanes in a city?

The other angle to consider in programme design is the overall aim, objectives or goal. This will help with deciding what method to use for evaluation (see Figure 8.5). There is a large range of methods that can be used to find information, but not every method is appropriate. Figure 8.5 gives an example of the 'type' of aim of a programme and the possible way to evaluate the achievement of this aim. For example, one way to measure behaviours is to evaluate behaviours in that context, for example, correct insulin injection use. Another example is the evaluation changes in policy that could be achieved by recording legislative changes locally or nationally. Remember that to be sure that an aim has been achieved, the evaluation chosen (or combination of methods chosen) has to measure the aim set. Evaluating knowledge of mobile phone theft safety measures

Objective	Possible method of evaluating
To change knowledge	Question and answer session
To change behaviour	Record data (e.g. number of clients now injected insulin correctly)
To change attitudes and values	Observe what a client says
To establish health-promoting environments	Measure pedestrian flows or number of green spaces
To enhance decision-making skills	Observe a demonstration in real-life situation
To change policy	Record legislative changes
To raise health awareness	Record number of people who took leaflets
To improve health status	Keep records of health indicators (e.g. blood pressure)

Figure 8.5   The link between objectives and methods of evaluation

by measuring the number of people that took a leaflet about mobile phone theft would not be an effective indicator of knowledge. You would need to ask the group questions about their knowledge, through perhaps question-and-answer sessions, questionnaires, short interviews or focus groups.

Activity 8.6:   Evaluation linked to aims of programmes

Using Figure 8.5 to help you, how might you measure the following?

1   Correct exercise techniques for a set of chair exercises in a fall-prevention group.
2   The successful establishment of a conservation programme in primary schools.
3   The correct technique for checking for lumps in testicular cancer.
4   The introduction of road traffic calming measures in a residential area.
5   To raise awareness of the risks of eating a diet high in saturated fats.

EVALUATION OF MASS COMMUNICATION

Mass communication in health that has been discussed in previous chapters is concerned with the sending of messages to the public without any personal contact. It may involve the use of mass media (for example, printed, audio visual and inter-active material) and the use of marketing strategies which seek to persuade people about health behaviours (Naidoo and Wills 2000). It has both strengths and weak-nesses. Its strengths lie in its ability to get messages to a wide audience, it is suc-cessful if simple messages are conveyed, and it can ensure that health issues are put on the public health agenda. Its weaknesses lie in the fact that it is rarely success-ful on its own, it doesn't convey complex messages well and can not teach skills or change attitudes or behaviours (Thorogood and Coombes 2004).

When attempting to evaluate mass communication it is important to recognize its significant limitations and to consider the use of models to assist in provid-ing a framework. If mass media is going to be effective, it is likely that it changes the way people view certain behaviours rather than changing the behaviour itself (Thorogood and Coombes 2004).

Activity 8.7:   Evaluation of mass communication

Use your knowledge of mass communication and how it works (for example from Chapter 4) to help you:

1   What do you think are the main problems with trying to evaluate mass communication?

Designing an evaluation process for mass communication should ensure a circular process, which begins with a formative research that should pre-test materials in order to limit the potential misinterpretation. Process evaluation is an essential tool in this area, as it needs to ask the questions of why it worked as well as it did, and can it uncover potential issues such as why did it not work?

EVALUATING THE DISSEMINATION OF RESULTS IN HEALTH PROMOTION

Dissemination of the findings in health promotion is an area that needs more development. If it is accepted that evaluation is a key component of any health promotion programme, it is essential that results be disseminated to the participants of the programme, the policy-makers and the practitioners. It helps to ensure that the findings are embedded in future policies and health behaviours. It is important to the building-up of a credible evidence base. It is also the right of all stakeholders to have access to the knowledge and potential benefits of the health intervention.

The benefits to disseminating evaluations of health promotion programmes are numerous and are outlined in Figure 8.6.

Benefits can be split into two categories, 'personal' and 'organizational'. Personal reasons for dissemination of evaluation findings includes wanting to search for meaning and understanding in work, to initiate change, or it may be an interest area for the practitioner. Organizational reasons to disseminate information include improving or promoting health, informing future policy and practice and responding to demands. Case Study 8.5 is an example of the use of evaluation for future work by the Stroke Association (2005).

Personal	Organizational
• Initiating change • Finding out • The search for meaning • The need to understand • Looking for causal relationships • Testing theories • Discovering the new • As part of a course or study • Specialist area of interest	• Improving health care and wellbeing • Planning for change and innovation • Informing policy and practice • Knowledge-based approach • Encouraging an evaluative culture • Responding to policies and demands • Reacting to public opinion • Delivering measurable results • Quality and audit • Cost effectiveness • Developing evidence-based practice

Figure 8.6   Personal and organizational reasons for evidence-based dissemination, adapted from Shober and Farrington (1998) with permission from Trent RDSU

Case Study 8.5   Stroke is a medical emergency

The Stroke Association's campaign 'Stroke is a medical emergency' is built on previous research and evaluation that found first that there is lack of awareness and misdiagnosis by health professionals, and second that the emergency services have an uncoordinated approach to stroke diagnosis and management. The campaign aims to address the lack of public awareness, misdiagnosis by health professionals and a lack of clear organizational structure to deal with stroke patients. The campaign was launched with the publication of a report *What's the emergency* (The Stroke Association 2005). One of the main messages is to diagnose a stroke acronym that can easily be remembered. 'FAST' is the assessment of three symptoms of stroke, known as the 'Face Arm Speech Test':

Facial weakness – can the person smile? Has their mouth or eye drooped?
Arm weakness – can the person raise both arms?
Speech problems – can the person speak clearly and understand what you say?
Test all three symptoms.

(Stroke Association 2005)

BARRIERS TO DISSEMINATING EVALUATION

Funding is not always considered when undertaking dissemination of findings. It is important when planning a health promotion programme that resources are allocated to this activity. From the perspective of an academic undertaking research, there is an expectation that they will publish their work, and this raises their credibility and status. The language of research is often complex and difficult for other people to understand. Access to the Internet should result in increased access to research findings; however, not everyone has access to this medium nor knows how to find what they are looking for.

Crosswaite and Curtice (1994) describe four ways in which findings are disseminated:

- *Rational*: it's enough to make the information available to be incorporated into policy.
- *Limestone*: research trickles into policy like water through limestone, for example, slowly and in a roundabout way.
- *Gadfly*: the emphasis is as much on the dissemination as it is on the research itself, so structures are put in place to make it happen.
- *Insider model*: researchers have links with governments or agencies and are able to adapt findings to suit.

The Gadfly model offers the best opportunity for achieving a satisfactory outcome as it concentrates its efforts on communicating messages to stakeholders. This could be in the form of written information, speaking to groups, arranging conferences, using the press and Internet or forming advisory groups.

Activity 8.8:   Dissemination of findings

Imagine that you are disseminating information with regard to the outcomes of a campaign to increase the use of a playgroup in an inner-city area of Bradford.

1   What types of communication could you employ to disseminate findings to the different target groups of users, policy-makers and practitioners?

It is important to remember that any dissemination of findings is not a one-way process. Feedback on the findings will continue to inform the evidence base and influence the way in which policies and practice are implemented. Mckee (2003) suggests that users should be trained in the process of evaluation to enable them to participate fully in framing questions and designing evaluation strategies. They should then be instrumental in assisting in the dissemination of findings along with professionals.

CONCLUSION

Evaluation skills are essential components of the health practitioner's portfolio, however, evaluating communication in health promotion is an area that requires further development. This is particularly pertinent in the light of developments in interactive media and access to the World Wide Web. Models of communication can be helpful in framing an evaluation strategy, particularly in the early stages of a programme, and their uses should be fully explored in future practice.

Methods used in assessing the impact of health programmes will always require a variety of ways that can demonstrate the complexity of how messages are received and interpreted. A combination of process, impact and outcome evaluation helps both researcher and stakeholder to engage in all aspects of the assessment of programme results. Evaluation should be commenced at the planning stage of any programme and carried on throughout. It is also important to remember when disseminating the evaluation findings, the means by which stakeholders obtain information and find ways in which the least empowered or influential are given the opportunity to access results, it is advantageous to disseminate findings not just for personal reasons but for alternative organization reasons as well.

Summary

- This chapter has examined the role of evaluation in health promotion through the exploration of evaluation theory in communication processes.
- Theoretical models of evaluation have been explored, including the well-known process, impact and outcome model, together with economic, pluralistic, participatory and social marketing evaluation techniques.
- This chapter has highlighted what could be measured through evaluation, including evaluation of mass media campaigns.
- Dissemination of evaluation findings has also been considered, and the rationale for engagement in this process.

ADDITIONAL READING

Two good general textbooks that cover a wider variety of areas around evaluation include:

Thorogood, M and Coombes, Y (eds) (2004) *Evaluating health promotion: practice and methods, 2nd edition.* Oxford University Press, Oxford.

Jones, L, Siddell, M and Douglas, J (eds) (2002) *The challenges of promoting health: exploration and action, 2nd edition.* Open University Press, Basingstoke.

Conclusion: Bridging theory and practice – ten different health promotion campaigns

Communicating health: strategies for health promotion has explored eight areas of communication in health promotion and health education practice. Now readers should be in a position to commence the design of communication strategies, to utilize methods and to undertake practice around communication design. This book concludes with ten different health promotion related campaigns to enable health practitioners to see models of good work in practice.

This section is designed to encourage exploration of the ten campaigns that have used a variety of strategies and methods to achieve their goals. They include many of the elements discussed in this textbook and embody the philosophy of promoting health in a number of ways, bringing together a variety of practitioners and ideas to achieve their aims. This is not a definitive list of health promotion campaigns, but is designed to encourage the reader to explore what works, and gain ideas and insights to inform their own practice. Although there are other campaigns that could have been chosen, these were selected because they are recent, cover a variety of audiences, topics and goals, and are accessible to the reader via the Internet. Health practitioners are encouraged to spend time looking at these campaigns via the websites provided to gain a final overview of how the theoretical concepts of this textbook are linked to practice.

1 THE USE OF THEORY IN HEALTH PROMOTION: 'NATIONAL NO SMOKING DAY'

National no smoking day is an annual event, where the charity campaigns to encourage people to make an attempt to quit on that day every year. Alongside a huge range of resources to advertise the event, there is guidance on the website for those wishing to quit. The website uses the transtheoretical model (see Chapter 1) to tailor information to different persons wanting to quit: pre-contemplation can access 'benefits of stopping', contemplation phases can access 'get ready to stop', action can view 'how to stop' and maintenance 'staying stopped'. View the website at www.nosmokingday.org.uk.

2 THE USE OF MULTI-MEDIA STRATEGIES IN HEALTH PROMOTION: 'DON'T PLAY THE SEX LOTTERY – USE A CONDOM'

The Department of Health (2005) launched the campaign 'Don't play the sex lottery – use a condom'. It was aimed at 18–30-year-olds and featured in lifestyle magazines, on the radio and in print media such as beer mats and scratch cards. A website and telephone helpline were also established. The website contains 'play the sex lottery' activities, including the one-armed bandit jackpot machine and 'gifts for lovers'. There is also a photo comic clinic visit with 'Gary' and an interactive postcode clinic finder. View the website at www.playingsafely.co.uk.

3 A CAMPAIGN TO COMPLIMENT POLICY CHANGES: 'KNOW WHAT YOU'RE GETTING INTO'

The Mayor of London and the Metropolitan Police are responsible for the campaign 'Know what you're getting into'. They have produced posters in a variety of locations, including pubs and clubs across London, with a short 'Safer travel at night' film. This is in response to London becoming a 24-hour city. There are a number of other policy improvements that support this campaign, including minicab licensing and night bus improvements. View the campaign at www.met.police.uk/sapphire/sapphire_minicabrape.htm.

4 A CAMPAIGN TIMED WITH A MAJOR EVENT: 'THINK! SUMMER DRINK DRIVE CAMPAIGN'

THINK! World Cup and summer drink drive campaign (DFTT 2006b) was aimed primarily at 17–29-year-old male drink (not drunk) drivers. The campaign incorporated a television advert 'crash' screened over the World Cup period alongside a cinema advert. There was also a radio advert, 'Nothing random', to support local police enforcement. For more information visit www.thinkroad-safety.gov.uk/campaigns.

5 A CAMPAIGN BASED ON A RESPONSE TO RESEARCH EVIDENCE: 'STROKE IS A MEDICAL EMERGENCY'

The Stroke Association's campaign 'Stroke is a medical emergency' is built on previous research and evaluation that found first that there is lack of awareness and misdiagnosis by health professionals, and second that the emergency services have an uncoordinated approach to stroke diagnosis and management. The campaign aims to address the lack of public awareness, misdiagnosis by health professionals and a lack of clear organizational structure to deal with stroke patients. The campaign was launced with the publication of the report *Stroke is a medical emergency* (Stroke Association 2005). To view more information visit www.strokeassociation.org.uk.

6 A CAMPAIGN TO ADVOCATE PUBLIC POLICY CHANGES: 'ARE WE TAKING THE DIS?'

The Disability Rights Commission (2006) is campaigning to change Britain and put disability at the heart of public policy. They propose 10 priorities for change, including increasing disabled people's participation, closing the employment gap, supporting independent living and promoting children's life chances. The 'Are we taking the dis?' campaign aims to highlight the inequity and inequalities experienced by those with a disability. 'I earn less than my collegues just for being deaf', or 'I'm a real fashion victim, I can't get into the shops' are just two of the advertising messages encouraging debates, forums and discussions around disability. You can view this at www.drc.org.uk/disabilitydebate.

7 A CAMPAIGN WITH INTERACTIVE RESOURCES TO ASSIST IN BEHAVIOUR CHANGE: 'SALT – EAT NO MORE THAN 6 G A DAY'

The Food Standards Agency (2006) salt reduction campaign 'Salt – eat no more than 6 g a day' aims to encourage people to reduce salt levels in their diet to no more than 6 g per day. This campaign was launched in 2005 and continues to use a variety of television and print media to promote a reduction in salt levels. The website contains a number of useful interactive resources to assist in behavioural change. These include how to check labels, a salt calculator, information on how to cook without salt, salt myths, a salt-o-meter and an 'Ask Sam' question forum. The website can be accessed at www.salt.gov.uk.

8 HEALTH PROMOTION VIA IT: 'TXT SAMARITANS 4 EMOTIONAL SUPPORT'

The Samaritains aim to make emotional health a mainstream issue. Their campaign methods include telephone calls, letters, emails and one-to-one work. Their latest campaigns are around promoting their 24/7 text support service for anyone in emotional distress. When a person sends a text message, they should receive a reply giving emotional support within ten minutes. View information about this campaign on www.samaritans.org.uk.

9 A CAMPAIGN TO PROVIDE INFORMATION: 'TALK TO FRANK'

'Talk to Frank' was established by the Department of Health for substance misuse information provision for young people and parents. There is a wealth of resources including the A–Z of drugs, quizzes (including a parents' quiz) and information giving resources and policies. The interactive elements available all aim to increase knowledge, for example, 'drag the drug onto the teenager to see the effect'. View the website at www.talktofrank.co.uk.

10 A CAMPAIGN DESIGNED TO CHANGE BEHAVIOUR: NHS 5-A-DAY

This NHS campaign aims to change behaviour so that everyone eats five pieces of fresh fruit and vegetables a day through multi media, including national television advertisments. The wesbite contains games, recipes, information for schools, parents and distributers/suppliers of fruit and vegetables. Resources include a wall chart, a portion poster, recipe booklets, postcard, leaflet and brochure, with information in a number of languages. There are area coordinators for regions of England to assist with the implementation of 5-a-day. View information about this campaign on www.5aday.nhs.uk.

Activity discussions

This section contains discussions from the activities throughout the textbook. They are designed not as definitive answers, but as suggested examples to the activities.

CHAPTER 1

1.1 How are health promotion messages communicated?

1 Traditional sources of communication such as television, radio, magazines, newspapers, Internet, telephone, one-to-one alongside more non-traditional sources such as sign language, symbols, text messages or eye contact.
2 Interpersonal information (one-to-one or group work) or different types of media including mass media (newspapers, magazines, television), print media (leaflets, booklets, posters), electronic media (Internet) and audio visual (radio, video).

1.2 Why not use theory?

1 Time, resources, finance, lack of expertise or difficulty of application to practice.

1.3 The role of wider determinants of health

1 Part funding from employers, national cycling schemes, school or work 'buddy' systems.
2 Use of after-school clubs, local groups such as Brownies, or youth groups might be able to provide supervision or local facilities.

1.4 The theory of planned behaviour in action

1 Yes, Daniel will probably take the steroids. Look again at Figure 1.5, and follow the format. He has a positive attitude (wants to look good) and a supportive subjective norm (a member of staff with 'muscles' already using steroids). Perceived behavioural control is more difficult; we are not sure if he is ready, willing and can access steroids, but will assume that he can. In regard of strong behavioural intention, all pointers indicate that he will try steroids to look good, resulting in the action of taking the steroids.

1.5 The health belief model in action

1   Suki will probably not take action on National No Smoking Day. Using Figure 1.6 as a guide, you can work through each stage of Suki's case study. In regard susceptibility/severity, her father has lung cancer and is in hospital; however, she does not regard herself as a smoker, and thus would probably not think she is susceptible. She has received a cue to action (National No Smoking Day information), although she may not feel the cue to action is appropriate to her as she is classing herself as a social smoker. Demographically we have to do a little guess-work: she smokes with alcohol after work, and her father is still alive, which suggests she is perhaps in the 18 to late 30s age bracket.

2   Suki cannot at this point in time see benefits to stopping (she does not think she is at risk). Hence the prediction will be that there is no action on National No Smoking Day.

1.6 The transtheoretical model in action

1   Maintaining.
2   Action.
3   Maintenance.
4   Pre-contemplation.
5   Readiness.
6   Contemplation.

1.7 The perceived behavioural control model in action

1   At the 'pre-knowledge' stage you would provide information or resources to move people to the 'knowledge' stage. At the 'knowledge' stage people would need to gain some knowledge about recycling and the facilities available. At the 'approval' stage people would agree that recycling bins are a good idea, and that recycling rubbish is a positive step. At the 'intention' stage, people would need to intend to recycle, for example, next time they have a collection of glass or paper. At the 'practice' stage people would be actively recycling their glass or paper. Finally, at the 'advocacy' stage they would be encouraging others to do the same.

1.8 The communication persuasion model in action

•   *Tuning in*: the person would be exposed to the message.
•   *Attending*: the person would have paid some attention to the message.
•   *Liking*: aspects (or all) of the message would be liked, for example, the people in it.
•   *Comprehend*: the message would be understood that condoms can prevent STIs.
•   *Generating*: the person will think about their own behaviours, and what they might have to do to use a condom.
•   *Acquiring*: the person will acquire skills, for example, purchasing condoms, correct usage of condoms.
•   *Agreeing*: the person needs to agree to use a condom at the next sexual encounter.
•   *Storing*: the person keeps the message for future use.
•   *Retrieval*: the person can recall the message in the next situation where a condom is required.
•   *Decision*: the person will make a decision to use condoms at the next situation where a condom is required.
•   *Acting*: the person will use a condom.
•   *Post action*: the person will continue to use a condom in all situations where a condom is required.
•   *Converting*: the person will advise or encourage others to use a condom.

1.9 Individual, structural or both?

1   Individual.
2   Combination of individual and structural.
3   Structural.

CHAPTER 2

2.1 Policies and practice

1   Examples include: Cancer – *The national cancer plan* (DOH 2000b);
    Physical activity – *Choosing health: making healthy choices easier* (DOH 2004); Older People –
    National service framework for older people (DOH 2001c).

2.2 Who gets priority?

Choosing health: making healthy choices easier (DOH 2004), priorities for action:

- Reducing number of people who smoke.
- Reducing obesity and improving diet/nutrition.
- Increasing exercise.
- Encouraging and supporting sensible drinking.
- Improving sexual health.
- Improving mental health.

1   b) and possibly a)
2   Examples include: other priorities, limited funds available for areas not allocated funding by
    some national policies, or the area is a target area.

2.3 Reactive or proactive

1   Reactive.
2   Reactive.
3   Proactive.
4   Both.
5   Both.

2.4 Differences in health behaviours

1   Different emphasis on preventive behaviours, including screening, and may have different health-
    related behaviours with regard to issues such as sexual health, safety or physical activity.
2   Different concerns; for example, females may have concerns around menopause or osteoporo-
    sis, whereas males may be more concerned with increased risks of prostate cancers or CHD.

2.5 Differences in communication

1   Different languages thus requiring different wording in one-to-one work. You might wish to
    address a message to 7-year-olds about brushing teeth regularly and correctly. Messages to 50-
    years-olds could focus on good dental hygiene, the importance of regular check-ups, or look-
    ing after sensitive teeth. The medium used may also be different; perhaps stickers or cartoons
    for 7-year-olds, information booklets for 50-year-olds.

2.6 Who is the message designed for?

1 Age: parents with children and upwards (note the symbol 'protect children').
2 Mixed sex.
3 Socio-economic: all inclusive, and the use of symbols and little writing mean the messages can reach groups who have limited literacy skills.
4 Education: little writing, few complex instructions and accessible to all groups.
5 Ethnicity: given the lack of writing and the use of symbols, this message could reach a range of ethnic groups who are at risk of sunburn.

2.7 Attitudes and complexity

1 *Positive*: they are a 'regular' jogger, which suggests they run frequently, and will not be adverse to rain. As they are age 35, this suggests some stability in attitudes.
2 *Both*: the 29-year-old has had a major health 'scare' at 29, and at their age they also have fairly stable attitudes. It is difficult to determine how much 'value' the 29-year-old will attach to a suntan.
3 *Negative*: they are 50, which suggest reasonably stable attitudes, and he has not been wearing a seatbelt for some time, so he will probably continue not to do so.

2.8 Attitudes, values and beliefs

1 Negative attitude to respiratory or skin problems, as he is using these hazards as part of his daily work.
2 He needs to use these substances to complete this daily work; he may believe that these substances do not harm him.
3 He may rate daily work highly (especially financial); he may rate health problems secondary to working.
4 Probably, unless there are other substances available, or the nature of the employment changes.

2.9 Campaigns to encourage positive attitudes

1 Examples include: 15–18-year-old white males at college; 60–80-year-old women, mixed ethnicity, attending dance classes; or 7–11-year-old school children in an after-school club.
2 A local role model, local sports personality, teacher, MP, older person's advocate or other.
3 This depends on the topic; breastfeeding could be 'breast is best' or recycling 'reduce, reuse, recycle'.
4 a) Case study 2 (MIND) suggests challenging stereotypes, one-to-one or small group work; b) the local setting could be school, workplace, hall, park etc.

CHAPTER 3

3.1 Defining hard-to-reach groups

1 Examples include: different ethnic groups, isolated older people, asylum seekers and refugees, homeless people, or those excluded from school.
2 Examples include: mainstream mass information sources may not be available, literacy skills may be low, low levels of self-esteem or social support and access to services is difficult.

3.2 Cultural identity

1   This is subjective and may centre on your own religious beliefs, behaviours or traditions among other factors.
2   Examples include: different beliefs than others, different attitudes, discriminatory, judgemental or discriminatory practices or inability to communicate in a different language.
3   Embrace diversity and difference, consider non-traditional ways of communicating or ensure adequate translation services are available.

3.3 Application of six principles of care

1   Examples include: discriminatory practices, not listening to others, not sharing information, not allowing two-way communication, disinterest, not allowing questions, not providing information in different formats or assuming dependency.

3.4 Overcoming barriers

1   Examples include: provide additional information resources (for example, leaflets or booklets), encourage talking between staff/patients and patient/patient, or allow time for questions.

3.5 Challenging the present

1   Aside from the last example, all of these involve contact between the user of the service and the provider of a service – either a mental-health-related service or other authority (i.e. police).
2   Projects could include: advocacy workers in these settings to encourage good communication, campaigns to reduce stigma of mental illness, promote understanding of different cultural beliefs around mental illness and mental health in the wider community, provide support for those identified as at risk, either emotional or resource based.

3.6 Communicating with older people

1   May prefer different information sources, and may have restricted access to sources. IT use may be limited in some groups. Different media sources (newspapers, magazines etc.) can be used as well as one-to-one communication, or print media (information booklets or leaflets).
2   Different preferences, particularly if using the classifications of young-old and old-old as detailed earlier in this chapter. There may be some cognitive, hearing or visual problems that restrict access to sources, and different methods should be used accordingly.

3.7 'Stop smoking' materials for those over 70

1   A large font would be preferable on written material, and use of audio materials should be considered. Use of an appropriate planning, implementation and evaluation framework should be used alongside the appropriate theoretical model.
2   No, and materials in this setting should use a combination of media.

3.8 'Healthy heart' programme design

1   Encourage heath professionals to make a referral to the class, telephone individuals, provide refreshments, offer one-to-one sessions alongside the group classes.
2   Making friends, appearance related or getting out of the house.
3   Website or telephone support.

3.9 NSF demonstrated outcomes

Example: Flu immunisation

1 A well-planned advertising campaign, letters from GP practices to all those at risk, provision of drop-in clinics (no appointments) to increase uptake.
2 Message design would focus on 'keeping well' in the winter, or keeping fit in the winter, the fact that it is easy to protect oneself, and free.

3.10 A new ambition and mental health

1 Age concern suggest that to improve mental health and wellbeing there are a number of things older age-groups can do. These include the addition of exercise in a daily routine, keeping the brain stimulated and maintaining a good work–life balance. See Age Concern's (2006) 'Top tips for maintaining good health' at www.ageconcern.org.uk.
2 Encourage the use of the Internet, use telephone support and use a 'buddy' system with local older people or a weekly club.

CHAPTER 4

4.1 Media in health promotion

1 There are hundreds of examples of media use in health promotion.
These might include the 'THINK!' UK government road safety adverts available at www.thinkroadsafety.gov.uk or the NHS 5-a-day campaign available at www.5aday.nhs.uk. Alternatively, they could include charity campaigns such as the 'SunSmart' campaign by Cancer Research available at www.cancerresearch.org.uk.
2 *Health behaviours*: those that encourage behaviour such as stopping smoking, or physical activity.
Risk reduction: those that aim to reduce risks, for example, sensible drinking, safe drug-taking or low cholesterol.
Health protection: those that promote vaccinations (for example, flu vaccines), testicular or breast screening.
Health education: those that contain educational messages, often found in stop-smoking messages (smoking is bad for your health) or HIV prevention (use a condom to prevent HIV).

4.2 Mass media and tobacco

1 The advantages of using media include widespread publicity, agenda-setting, reaches the whole population, counteracts the pro-smoking lobby, opportunistic, the message that tobacco is a major public health issue. There is limited evidence that mass media is effective using these examples, and is not suitable for all groups; it could give mixed messages, and will not appeal and reach all groups.
2 One-to-one, skills-based group work, early-school-based education (primary), social marketing strategies may be effective and lobbying the pro-tobacco groups for change (see www.ash.org.uk for more information on lobbying).

4.3 Suitability of methods for mass media

1 Remember that the media cannot teach skills or change strong attitudes. There is a possibility that a) and b) could be achieved through mass media.

2   a) Raising awareness could be achieved via mass media publicity materials.
    b) As with a), mass media could use publicity to advertise a new telephone service.
    c) Mass media could provide awareness of a service, but cannot directly increase rates of those screened.
    d) Mass media cannot provide skills.
    e) Mass media cannot change strong attitudes, but it may influence these (see Case Study 3, Chapter 2).
    Alternative methods include skills-based-work and interactive resources that allow active learning.

4.4 Supportive environments – environments and economics

1   a) Opportunistic health promotion, including after-school clubs, parks or sports centres.
    b) Free loan or renting schemes, discount vouchers for use in local shops.
    c) Preventive measures at other opportunities, for example, a person attending a pharmacy or shopping centre where 'mobile' screening units might be available.
    The roles of advocacy or lobbying might be necessary to make these areas priorities.

4.5 A sensible drinking campaign message

1   Sensible *drinking* words might include: responsibility, stopping at too much, saying 'no'. *18–25* words can include: young adults, youth or students. Motivations to *'drink sensibly'* can include: unwanted pregnancy, accidents, appearance, not being sick, embarrassment, morning after.
2   An example could be: 'students', 'knowing your limit', 'unwanted pregnancy'.
3   A slogan based on the premise of sticking to a limit, and not experiencing unwanted pregnancy, or emergency contraception could be 'Remember the night before and forget the morning after'.

4.6 Message placement

1   As the designed message from Activity 5 was aimed at students, the message could be displayed in a university setting, including the student union, toilets, halls of residence or around the university environment, for example local pharmacies or pubs.

4.7 Audience segmentation

1   Groups can include secondary school children, those in a workplace, church-goers, youth groups or young parents.
2   An example setting is a workplace. The group can be split into male/female, sexual preference (homosexual/heterosexual), contraceptive users/non-contraceptive users, high risk/low risk and so on, to allow accurate targeting of messages.

4.8 The 4 Ps

1   *Product:* salt (added to food, added in cooking, already in foods).
    Price: this can be actual costs (salt is cheap), like the taste, habit to add to cooking and so on.
    Place: Buy food in the supermarket and cook at home, so any placement of a message should probably be in either of these locations.
    Promotion: want to look at reducing salt to current government recommendations (6 g) (see www.salt.gov.uk).
    Positioning: a message in the supermarket; a message on the salt container; a message in the home that appeals to the proposed target group.

4.9 Local newspapers

1   Could include human interest stories, a chat column, advertising events, or press releases.

4.10 Media advocacy

1   Tobacco companies, fast-food manufacturers, non-fair-trade companies or large manufacturers who have lax working or employment laws.
2   An example is tobacco: you can draw attention to the risks of smoking, use case studies to highlight the 'people's' angle, find statistical evidence, use local groups and coalitions or protest and lobby local MPs or local organizations.

4.11 Fear appeals

1   Risks include: loss of memory, inability to function normally, physical or sexual assault and black-outs.
2   Messages can include: keep your drink with you at all times, only accept drinks from people you know, or do not accept drinks you are unsure about or that taste unusual.

CHAPTER 5

5.1 How could IT be used to ...?

1   Mobile phones, Internet quizzes, email or touch-screens.
2   Email, Internet, chat rooms, interactive software (i.e. CD-ROMs) or computer games.

5.2 Interactive websites

1   A variety of government, organizational and commercial websites.
2   Websites can contain interactive resources such as alcohol unit calculators, smoking calculators, BMI calculators, diaries, chat rooms, games, activities and quizzes.

5.3 Touch-screen kiosks

1   It is already in the GP centre where patients have come for consultations; it is next to other health information; possible low IT skills of users; there are no prompts from staff or information signs; it is located in a public space and patients may have no time.
2   Staff could promote its use; it could be clearly signposted; placed in a more private location; or GPs could prompt use after the consultation.

5.4 SMS messaging services

1   Sexual health messages; some test results; simple information such as appointment reminders; short motivating messages (mental health or physical activity).
2   Complex information; behaviour change information; anything regarded as unwanted information.

5.5 Designing a website

1   Health and hygiene, employment and benefit advice, sources of advice, maintaining positive mental health or information around risky behaviours.

2 As target groups are mixed and it is difficult to identify one single type of user, information should be simple, straightforward and jargon-free, easy to read and navigate, and available in different languages.
3 Free Internet access at shelters, libraries, job centres, supermarkets or other locations that this group may access.

5.6 Tailoring messages

1 *Precontemplation*: general information-giving, with advice number if help needed in the future.
Contemplation: appealing to current motivations, for example, losing weight before a holiday or big event.
Readiness: how to achieve goals, for example, which trainers to buy, which gym class to choose or which nights of the week for walking.
Action: advice on keeping going with exercise, tips for low motivation, and positive reinforcement of messages.
Maintenance: positive reinforcement.

5.7 Health belief model barriers on a website

1 These include cost, habit, taste, price, access, culture, not knowing how to cook, time or children not liking healthy foods.
2 Messages could centre on 'easy' cooking, low prices, sauces and dressings to add variety and taste, and child friendly meals.

5.8 The seven-step checklist for a website design

An example of website design for this group includes:

1 Challenging attitudes and beliefs suggests that an interactive element is necessary, perhaps including quizzes, a chat room, fashion tips or a 'reader's email corner'.
2 Someone who embodies positive body image and who is of the average size female. A health professional may be helpful in answering reader's emails.
3 Ones that embody feeling good about one's self.
4 Colourful, informative and encouraging 'sharing' of information.
5 Quizzes, a chat room or a 'reader's email corner'.
6 Enable anonymous emails.
7 Anywhere where this age group might be found, including university, workplaces, women's groups or other organizations.

5.9 Practical barriers

1 Access in different locations, need for large screens or audio or spoken word for those with visual impairment.
2 Selecting different locations or using locations differently, for example, 'women only' Internet cafés. Helpers could be available in some locations to assist with any visual/audio problems, make headphones available if sounds needed. Provide information in different formats.

5.10 Recommending websites

1 Ask yourself questions such as: Is it a reputable organization? Does the site have a wide range of information? Is it is easy to access? Is the organization trustworthy? What sort of organization is it? Is the information jargon-free? Is there any interpersonal contact?

CHAPTER 6

6.1 Types of settings for different target groups

Example target group: Primary school children, 5–11 years.

1 Schools, after-school clubs, activity clubs, local community.
2 Mixed or competing messages, parental control, different aims of teachers or the school's governing bodies.

6.2 Fitting activities to setting-based models

1 Organic.
2 Vehicle.
3 Active.
4 Comprehensive.
5 Passive.

6.3 Traditional and non-traditional settings

1 *Educational*: schools, higher education, universities or pre-school.
   Health care: primary care, hospitals, dentists or NHS walk-in centres.
   Social: supermarkets, pubs or workplaces.
2 *Traditional*: are widely used, including schools, hospitals, neighbourhoods, workplaces. *Non-traditional*: those that are not as widely used, including universities, barber shops, hairdressers, travel agents or churches.

6.4 Overcoming disadvantages of settings

1 Manpower could involve community or voluntary groups; resources could make use of the wider community and its facilities. Reaching excluded groups will entail choosing different settings, and to include environmental and social aspects, a holistic notion of health will need to be embodied in the whole programme.

6.5 Designing messages for a religious group

1 Any religious group could be chosen. Resources can include leaflets or posters with spiritual messages, biblical quotes on materials to encourage healthy behaviours, a prize quiz about aspects of health, competitions, a new website, SMS text messages or other interactive resources.

6.6 Designing healthy university resources

1 Use appropriate age messages with a catchy theme, show 'student-style' foods, for example pasta or pulses, promote ways to eat more healthily on small budgets.
2 Students will turn into the educators for the future generation, role of education in health, many health opportunities, large body of students and organizations.

6.7 Using barbers or beauty salons

Example: Barbers.

1   Sexual health, CHD risk, diabetes, prostate cancer, testicular cancer and other areas of high risk.
2   Poor evidence base, so the target group will need to be in close consultation with the project. Access might be difficult and the setting will need to provide a range of opening hours. Limited resources or manpower will mean that involving the wider community is essential.

6.8 Opportunistic settings use and travel health

1   This could be designed with a range of 'themed words' (as in Activity 4.5). Loss, annoyance, difficulties, financial problems and so on could form the core of the message design, and thus 'keep your wallet safe when walking', or 'lock your luggage', might be key theft prevention messages.
2   This message could be on the back of airline or rail tickets, on travel websites, in aeroplane magazines, in apartments and hotels or other places where travellers are likely to be.

CHAPTER 7

7.1 Evidence-based practice rationale

1. Evidence embodies the ideals of good practice, it ensures inclusivity and that no-one is excluded or discriminated against. It enables structured working, ensures cooperation, you can help predict any unplanned effects or additional resources and minimise risk of failures.

7.2 What evidence do you use?

1   Community-based work might use 2, 3 and 4. Clinical practice is most likely to use 1 and 2. Students in subjects such as research methods will probably examine the upper of these levels, health policy or local planning might use the lower levels.

7.3 Planning with evidence

1   You could undertake a small pilot study using the council solution (community police officers). You could set up a project that expands on existing projects, for example include 'youths' in this. You could also approach the 'youths' and see what they might want.
2   You should examine other projects in similar neighbourhoods that aim to reduce crime, for example 'New deal for community' (NDC) projects or 'Healthy cities' projects.

7.4 NICE evidence base

1   Their website contains a variety of policy documentation, best practice, evidence-based briefings and other guidelines for good practice.

7.5 Grey literature

1   You could use health impact assessments (HIA), needs assessments, community profiles, annual reports, minutes of meetings, informal and formal local project reports.
2   You may have been involved in compiling any of these, alongside your more formal work.

7.6 Including developing countries

1 Problems can include: difficulties in representing those with little power; may not be able to reach all of those who should be represented; resource and financial implications; and poor or corrupt management.
2 Suggestions include: start small; try to maintain a base of local projects that can be accessed at national and international level; encourage project leaders to report findings and record these; hold conferences 'on site' rather than in high-class locations; and delegate time and space to listening to others.

7.7 Acceptability and transferability

1 *Applicability criteria indicates*:

- There are few potential barriers.
- The group have expressed an interest so there may be only minor problems in acceptance.
- Contents can be tailored to the new sample; ethnicity shows some similarities.
- There are limited resources so involvement of the women's groups is essential.
- There may be some non-engagement problems.
- The organization running the project is similar (health-promotion focussed); barriers might include money or language.
- There is a professional physical activity coordinator available, although with a slightly different previous focus.

Transferability criteria indicates:

- There will be a need to investigate prevalence; general statistics indicate approximately 1 in 3 women are at risk.
- Some similarities, the women are close in age; there may be some psychological factors that are different, for example, perceived susceptibility and severity.
- Capacity is less in the target setting, and some activities may have to be tailored or adapted – perhaps a shortened programme or different delivery structures.

2 To ensure more success you could involve women's groups in the planning and provision of the programme; consider a pilot study first, and materials may need to be translated.

7.8 Evidence and smoking cessation

Example 1: Advice and support in community, primary and secondary care. A project based on this could be the provision of advice and training for pharmacists, dentists or physiotherapists to provide advice and support for those who want to stop smoking.
Example 2: Sensitive, and tailored to individuals. A project could use the transtheoretical model (see Chapter 1) on a website to encourage people to place themselves at stages of change, and match information resources accordingly to that stage.

CHAPTER 8

8.1 Who is interested in evaluation?

1 All of these headings might be appropriate reasons to evaluate this programme.
2 The local business community, for example, the chamber of commerce. The primary health care team, including health visitors, midwives and GPs. Voluntary groups, including the National Childbirth Trust or different women's groups. The local council, playgroups and nurseries, local MP or the local press.

8.2 Using process, impact and outcome evaluation

1   Examples include:
    Process: a comparison between one-to-one support and group sessions, what were the motivations for participants giving up, for example health, economy and peer pressure.
    Impact: the number of people who gave up in a given period or the number that reduced their consumption.
    Outcome: how many participants had taken up smoking again in one year.

8.3 Participatory evaluation in action

1   Examples include: keeping a photo diary of a vegetable growing in the garden; writing a story about a vegetable character; using songs and rhymes about the 5-a-day message; holding a harvest festival.

8.4 Validity in evaluation

1   *Internal validity*: in this example you will need to know the starting points of the programme, such as weight, type of exercise and diet undertaken. In this scenario you are not comparing like with like, so you would need to think about control groups; how would you know, for instance, that the dietary group were not taking additional exercise?
    External validity: you may need to exclude variables such as occupation, ethnicity, age, or social norms of the groups.
2   Examples include: having a control group, testing pre/post groups, taking into consideration wider variables (for example other projects) and pre-testing measurement instruments.

8.5 Ways to evaluate health communication

1   Examples include:
    Accuracy: were the key messages about using cycle paths clear and unambiguous, backed by factual information?
    Availability: was the information available in schools, work places, GP surgeries? What methods were used for publicity, i.e. newspapers, local radio?
    Balance: were the messages about the benefits of using cycle paths supported by advice such as personal safety or wearing a helmet?
    Consistency: were the messages about health benefits clear and unambiguous? Did the messages change during the campaign?
    Cultural competency: was consideration given to target groups across age, gender and ethnicity? How were the messages adapted to meet these needs?
    Evidence base: were any claims for physical or psychological benefits based on reliable studies? Did the campaign show evidence that there had been user consultation and involvement across a wide range of people?
    Reach: were hard to reach groups engaged? Were there incentives built into the programme, such as bicycle offers, competitions or bicycle lessons?
    Reliability: was there evidence of robust planning processes which had considered the most effective strategies for the campaign?
    Repetition: was there evidence that the key messages were user-friendly and easily remembered? Were the key messages reinforced across a variety of media?

8.6 Evaluation linked to aims of programmes

Often a combination of evaluation is suggested rather than one type of evaluation. Examples include:

1   Demonstration of three correct chair exercises. Number of people pre/post, who can successfully complete the programme of exercises.
2   Number of children involved in the programme. Correct identification of three types of species being conserved in the project, i.e. insects.
3   Question and answer session about correct technique. Short 'do you do the following' quiz on a website.
4   Survey to see if local residents think cars are slower (pre/post test this group). Reduction in accidents over a pre/post period.
5   Correct identification of high-fat foods through a questionnaire. Number of people pre/post who buy reduced-fat option foods.

8.7 Evaluation of mass communication

1   There is no way of knowing if the intended audience is being reached, therefore it is difficult to know if the message has reached the right people. It may reach the wrong audience and have no effect or be misinterpreted. It is difficult to obtain feedback and observed results may be diminished due to large numbers or results may not be attributable just to mass media.

8.8 Dissemination of findings

1   Examples include:
    Users: a visit to the playgroup to talk to parents and playgroup leaders, leaflets left in GP surgeries or in child health clinics.
    Policy-makers: presentations at council meetings, local health authority or primary care trusts, or post articles on well-accessed Internet sites or intranets.
    Practitioners: Publish articles on health promotion websites, attend team meetings of health care practitioners including GPs, health visitors or health promotion team. Disseminate information via formal research networks.

Glossary

Agenda setting Refers to the way the media select events that the public sees and with this selection set the terms of reference for current interest and debate.

At-risk groups A group that is vulnerable or susceptible to 'risk' of different types of ill health or disease.

Attitudes An evaluation that a person makes about an attitude 'object'. The attitude 'object' could be themselves, other people, issues (i.e. in the media) or objects (i.e. alcohol).

Beliefs The information that a person has about an object or action forms their beliefs.

Bottom-up approach This proposes that communities or groups know what they want and are involved in all stages of planning and implementing interventions (see Top-down approach).

Brief interventions A short health promotion session (i.e. 15 minutes) that is designed to prompt behaviour change or challenge attitudes to health-related behaviour.

Bus wraps A large bill-board style message placed on the outside of a bus.

Campaign A planned, designed and coordinated effort to promote a particular cause.

Chat rooms An Internet-based portal where anyone can 'chat' to each other via a mechanism similar to email.

Coercive communication usually a policy, law or rule enforced by the influential figures to stop a behaviour or action, often through legislation or peer pressure, i.e. not smoking in a public place.

Communication–persuasion model An input–output matrix that can be used to predict the levels a person will need to go through to achieve a behavioural change.

Demographics The characteristics of the population (i.e. social class, age or education) that can be measured via population groups.

Discrimination The placement of a person below that of another person who does not share the same characteristics (i.e. ethnic group or sex).

E-health A generic term for all IT applications linked to health and incorporating applications linked to computers, health and medicine that are used to deliver or promote health.

Empathy This is the ability of a health practitioner to place themselves in another's position and identify or understand what they have experienced and felt.

Empowerment A term usually used to describe a way of working that enables people to develop knowledge or skills to increase control and power over life circumstances.

Equity In health equity is concerned with the differences in health status that are unfair or unequal and the readdressing of these.

Evaluation The process by which worth or value of something is decided involving measurement, observation and comparison with the programme/policy aim.

Evidence-based practice The use of research evidence to guide practice.

Gaming The use of technology (i.e. mobile phones or internet) for game playing purposes. In health promotion these can be games with educational messages or interactions that challenge current practices or enforce current behaviours.

Health advocacy A combination of individual and social actions designed to gain political commitment, support or acceptance.

Health belief model A model of behavioural change that focuses on an individual weighing up the risks and benefits of behaviour.

Health Development Agency (HDA) A UK-based specialist health authority that aimed to improve the health of people in England. It has now closed, and has been partly replaced by NICE (see NICE).

Health education Providing information through constructed opportunities that improve knowledge or skills and increase healthy behaviours.

Health promotion The process of enabling people to increase control over their health.

Hierarchy of need A model which has five stages that can be used for understanding motivation. Each stage has to be satisfied before moving to the next stage, from physiological needs to self-actualization.

Holism Embodying holistic notions of health (see Holistic).

Holistic A term that includes the wider definition of health including physical, mental, social and spiritual health.

Inequalities (in health) Differences in health status between populations or sections of the population.

IT – Information technology, generally includes all interactive media (i.e. CD-ROMs, the Internet, touch-screen kiosks or computers).

Mass media Any type of printed or electronic communication medium that is sent to the population at large.

Model A simplified version of a theoretical construct.

Morbidity The amount of disease there is in a population (i.e. the number of people living with a disease).

Mortality The number of people who have died in the population (i.e. the number of people who have died from certain diseases).

National Service Framework(s) The UK government's long-term strategies for improving different areas of care (i.e. mental health).

NICE – The National Institute for Health and Clinical Excellence, the UK's independent health-related organization responsible for providing national guidance on the promotion, prevention and treatment in health.

Ottawa Charter for Health Promotion   A World Health Organization policy statement that sets out a clear commitment to health promotion.

Peer education   An education method where a person or group with credibility (i.e. older children) work with others (i.e. younger children) to promote health or prevent ill health.

Perceived behavioural control   Theoretical model that postulates behaviour can change through a series of steps.

Persuasive communication   A message that uses enticing or persuading techniques to encourage a change or modification in behaviour, attitudes or beliefs.

Prevention   The avoidance of hazards or risks through the creation of conditions to help avoidance or promote early detection of the hazard or risk.

Prosodic   The vocal intonation or rhythmatic aspects of language including pitch or stress placed on words.

Process of behaviour change   A step-based model based on the stages a person goes through when making a change in their behaviour.

Public health   A societal effort to prevent disease and prolonging life.

Role play   An education method where a person 'acts' a response to a situation (i.e. saying 'no' to cigarettes). The audience will then 'model' this same response in a real-life situation.

Screening   The procedure for the identification of a certain disease (i.e. breast cancer) to enable early detection and treatment of the disease.

Self-efficacy   An individual's judgement of their ability to achieve a certain goal (i.e. stopping smoking).

Settings-based approach   Any of a number of locations where people work, play and learn where health can be promoted.

SMS messaging   'Short messaging service', the facility and sending of short messages via a mobile phone, more commonly called 'text messaging'.

Stereotyping   The act of predicting how another person will act or behave in a certain situation based on preconceived notions of how people act (see Discrimination).

Tailoring information   Adapted information for a specific group of people to fit their needs and preferences.

Theory   A set of ideas or arguments that help to understand behaviour in a more simplified way.

Theory of planned behaviour   A theoretical model based on the stages a person goes through when changing a behaviour, including perceived behavioural control.

Theory of reasoned action   A theoretical model based on the stages a person goes through when changing behaviour; this model is a recent revision of the theory of planned behaviour model.

Top-down approach   An approach which is dictated by those with power that does not directly include the target group or receivers of the intervention (see Bottom-up approach).

Transtheoretical model or 'stages of change' model   A stage-step model based on the stages people go through when making a change in their behaviour.

UNICEF   The United Nations Children's Fund, which has 37 committees world-wide working with, and for, the world's children.

Values   Acquired by the social world, they can influence attitudes and behaviour.

References

Aaron, K F, Levine, D & Burstin, H (2003) African American church participation and health care practices. *Journal of General Intern Medicine* 18, 908–913

Abraham, C, Krahe, B, Dominic, R & Fritsche, I (2002) Do health promotion messages target cognitive and behavioural correlates of condom use? A content analysis of safer sex promotion leaflets in two countries. *British Journal of Health Psychology* 7 (2) 227–246

Acheson, D (1998) *Independent inquiry into inequalities in health.* The Stationery Office, London

Action for Health & Senior Citizens in Newcastle (1996) *The links to a fuller life.* Healthy City Project, Newcastle upon Tyne

Age Concern (2006) *Living room,* available at www.ageconcern.org.uk

Airhihenbuwa, C O & Obregon, R (2000) A critical assessment of theories/models used in health communication for HIV/AIDS. *Journal of Health Communication* 5 (Suppl.) 5–15

Ajzen, I & Fishbein, M (1980) *Understanding attitudes and predicting social behaviour.* Prentice-Hall, New Jersey

Ajzen (1991) The theory of planned behaviour. *Organisational Behaviour and Human Decision Processes* 50 179–211, available at www.unix.oit.umass.edu/~aizen/index.html

Alcalay, R & Bell, R (2000) Promoting nutritional physical activity through social marketing: current practice and recommendations. Centre for Advanced Studies in Nutrition and Social Marketing, University of California, available at www.socialmarketingnutrition.ucdavis.edu/downloads/alcalaybell.pdf

Andrews, A, Jeffels, S, Khan, A A & Weller, P (1995) Places of worship as settings for health promotion. Pilot research and development project. Religious studies subject area, University of Derby, available at www.multifaithnet.org

Arber, S & Ginn, J (1995) *Connecting gender and ageing: a sociological approach.* Open University Press, Buckingham

Ashbridge, M (2006) Public place restrictions on smoking in Canada: assessing the role of the state, media, science and public health advocacy. *Social Science and Medicine* 58 (1) 13–24

Atkin, C (2001) Theory and principles of media health campaigns, pp. 49–68 in Rice, R E & Atkin, C K (eds) Public communication campaigns, 3rd edition. Sage, London

Atun, R A, Samyshkin, Y, Thomas, L, McKee, M, Sittampalam, S & Coker, R (2006) The potential of SMS applications for the control of tuberculosis. *The Vodafone Policy Paper Series.* 4 (March), 29–38 available at www.vodafone.com

Atun, R A & Sittampalam, S R (2006) A review of the characteristics and benefits of SMS in delivering health care. *The Vodafone Policy Paper Series.* 4 (March) 18–28, available at www.vodafone.com

Austin, E W (1995) Reaching young audiences: developmental considerations in designing health messages, pp. 114–145 in Maibach, E & Parrott, R L (1995) *Designing health messages.* Sage, London

Baker, A & Macpherson, B (2000) Tomorrow's minds. MIND, London, available at www.mind.org.uk

Barbour, T, Caetano, R, Casswell, S, Edwards, G, Giesbrecht, N, Graham, K, Giube, J, Gruenewald, P, Mill, L, Holdes, M, Homel, R, Osterberg, E, Rehm, J, Roan, R, & Rossow, I (2003) *Alcohol – no ordinary commodity.* World Health Organisation/Society for Addiction, WHO, London

Baric, L (1993) The setting approach – implications for policy and strategy. *Journal of the Institute of Health Education* 31 (1) 17–24

Bates, C, McIntyre, D & Watt, T (2003) How to run a national tobacco campaign. ASH, available at www.ash.org.uk

Bauer, I L (2002) Travel advice as recalled by 522 tourists to Peru. *Journal of Travel Medicine* 9 (6) 293–396

Becker, M H (1974) The health belief model and personal health behaviour. *Health Education Monographs* 2 (4) 324–473

Beiner, L, Reimer, R L, Wakefield, M, Szczypka, G, Rigotti, N A & Connolly, G (2006) Impact of smoking cessation and mass media among recent quitters. *American Journal of Preventive Medicine* 30 (3) 217–224

Benigeri, M & Pluye, P (2003) Shortcomings of health information on the Internet. *Health Promotion International* 18 (4) 381–386

Benjamins, M R & Brown, C (2004) Religion and preventive health care utilization among the elderly. *Social Science and Medicine* 58, 109–118

Bennett, P & Murphy, S (1997) *Psychology and health promotion*. Open University Press, Buckingham

Bensberg, M & Kennedy, M (2002) A framework for health promoting emergency departments. *Health Promotion International* 17 (2) 179–188

Berger, M, Wagner, T H & Baker, L C (2005) Internet use and stigmatised illness. *Social Science and Medicine* 68 (8) 1821–1827

Bessinger, R, Katende, C & Gupta, N (2004) Multi-media campaign exposure effects on knowledge and use of condoms for STI and HIV/AIDS prevention in Uganda. *Evaluation and Program Planning* 27, 397–407

Bledsoe, L (2005) Smoking cessation; an application of theory of planned behaviour to understanding progress through stages of change. *Addictive Behaviours* 30 (7) 1335–1341

Boudioni, M (2003) Availability and use of touch-screen kiosks (to facilitate social inclusion). *Aslib Proceedings* 55 (5/6) 320–333, available at www.emeraldinsight.com

Brug, J, Conner, M, Harré, N, Kremers, S, McKeller, S & Whitelaw, S (2005) The transtheoretical model of change: a critique. *Health Education Research* 20 (2) 244–258

Bull, S S, McFarlane, M & King, D (2001) Barriers to STD/HIV prevention on the Internet. *Health Education Research* 16 (6) 661–670

Buller, D B, Woodhall, W G, Hall, J R, Borland, R, Ax, B, Brown, M & Hines, J M (2001) A web-based smoking cessation and prevention program for children aged 12–15, pp. 357–372 in Rice, R E & Aktin, C K (eds) (2001) *Public communication campaigns*, 3rd edition. Sage, California

Bunton, R & Macdonald, G (2002) *Health Promotion: Disciplines, diversity and developments* 2nd edition. Taylor & Francis: London

Burns, M E, See Tai, S, Lai, R & Nazareth, I (2006) Interactive health communication applications for people with chronic disease (review). *The Cochrane Library* Issue 1, available at www.thecochrane library.com

Byrd, T L, Peterson, S K, Chavez, R & Heckert, A (2004) Cervical screening beliefs among young Hispanic women. *Preventive Medicine* 38 (2) 192–197

Campbell, M K, James, A, Hudson, M A, Carr, C, Jackson, E, Oates, V, Demissie, S, Farrell, D & Tessaro, I (2004) Improving multiple behaviours for colorectal cancer prevention among African American church members. *Health Psychology* 23 (5) 492–502

Cancer Research (2006) *Be SunSmart*, available at www.cancerresearch.org.uk

Cashen, M S, Dykes, P & Gerber, B (2004) Ehealth technology and Internet resources. Barriers for vulnerable population. *Journal of Cardiovascular Nursing* 19 (3) 209–214

Cassell, M M, Jackson, C & Cheuvront, B (1998) Health communication on the Internet: an effective channel for behaviour change? *Journal of Health Communication* 3 (1) 71–79

Cavill, N, Buxton, K, Bull, F & Foster, C (2006) *Promotion of physical activity among adults, evidence into practice briefing*. HDA, London, available at www.publichealth.nice.org.uk

Centre for Communication Programmes (CCP) (2003) *A field guide to designing a health communication strategy*. Johns Hopkins University, available at www.jhuccp.org

Chew, F, Palmer, S, Slonska, Z & Jubbiah, S (2002) Enhancing health knowledge, health beliefs and health behaviour in Poland through a health promoting television program series. *Journal of Health Communication* 7 (3) 179–196

Christensen, C L, Bowen, D J, Hart, A, Kuniyuki, A, Saleeba, A E & Kramish Campbell, M (2005) Recruitment of religious organisations into a community-based health promotion programme. *Health and Social Care in the Community* 13 (4) 313–322

Cline, R J W & Hayes, K M (2001) Consumer health information seeking on the Internet: the state of the art. *Health Education Research* 16 (6) 671–692

Cohen, D A, Scribner, R A, & Farley T A (2000) A structural model of health behaviour: a pragmatic approach to explain and influence health behaviours at the population level. *Preventive Medicine* 30 (2) 146–154

Comm, C L & Mathaisel, D F X (2003) Less is more: a framework for a sustainable university. *International Journal of Sustainability in Higher Education* 4 (4) 314–323

Cooper, C P, Roter, D L & Langlieb, A M (2000) Using entertainment television to build a context for prevention news stories. *Preventive Medicine* 31 (3) 225–231

Cornwall and the Isles of Scilly Health Authority (1999) Bones in Mind osteoporosis project. Cornwall and IOS HP Department, Cornwall

Crosswaite, C & Cuitice, L (1994) Disseminating research results – The challenge of bridging the gap between health research and health action. *Health promotion international* 9 (4) 289–296

Cumming, E & Henry, W E (1961) *Growing old.* Basic Books, New York

Cummins, S & Macintyre, S (2002) 'Food deserts' – evidence and assumptions in health policy making. *British Medical Journal* 325, 436–438

Davis, S, Edmister, J, Sullivan, K & West, C (2003) Educating sustainable societies for the twenty-first century. *International Journal of Sustainability in higher education* 4 (2) 169–179

De Nooijer, J, Lechner, L, de Vries, H (2002) Tailored versus general information on early detection of cancer: a comparison of the reactions of Dutch adults and the impact on attitudes and behaviours. *Health Education Research* 17 (2) 239–252

De Wit, J B F, Vef, R, Schutten, M & Van Steenbergen, J (2005) Social-cognitive determinants of vaccination behaviour against hepatitis B: an assessment among men who have sex with men. *Preventive Medicine* 40 (6) 795–802

Demiris, G, Edison, K & Vijaykumar, S (2005) A comparison of communication models of traditional and video-mediated health care delivery. *International Journal of Medical Informatics* 74 (10) 851–856

Department for Education & Skills (DfES) (2004a) *Every child matters.* The Stationery Office, London

Department for Education & Skills (DfES) (2004b) *Healthy living blueprint for schools.* The Stationery Office, London

Department for Transport (2006a) *Think! Hedgehogs road safety campaign,* available at www.hedge-hogs.gov.uk

Department for Transport (2006b) *THINK! World Cup and summer drink drive campaign,* available at www.thinkroadsafety.gov.uk/campaigns

Department of Health (1992) *The health of the nation.* HMSO, London

Department of Health (1999) *Saving lives: our healthier nation.* The Stationery Office, Norwich, available at www.dh.gov.uk

Department of Health (2000a) *The NHS plan: a plan for investment – a plan for reform.* HMSO, London, available at www.dh.gov.uk

Department of Health (2000b) *The national cancer plan.* HMSO, London, available at www.dh.gov.uk

Department of Health (2001a) *Race equality in the Department of Health: race relations (amendment) act 2000.* The Stationery Office, Norwich, available at www.dh.gov.uk

Department of Health (2001b) *The expert patient: a new approach to chronic disease management for the 21st century.* The Stationery Office, Norwich, available at www.dh.gov.uk

Department of Health (2001c) *National service framework for older people.* The Stationery Office, London, available at www.dh.gov.uk

Department of Health (2002) *Health promoting prisons: a shared approach.* Stationery Office, London, available at www.dh.gov.uk

Department of Health (2003) *Effective sexual health promotion.* Stationery Office, London, available at www.dh.gov.uk

Department of Health (2004) *Choosing health: making healthy choices easier.* The Stationery Office, London, available at www.dh.gov.uk

Department of Health (2005) *Playing safely,* available at www.playingsafely.co.uk

Department of Health (2006a) *A new ambition for old age: next steps in implementing the national service framework.* The Stationery Office, London, available at www.dh.gov.uk

Department of Health (2006b) *Our health, our care, our say: a new direction for community services.* Stationery Office, London

Department of Health (2006c) *Talk to Frank,* available at www.talktofrank.com

DiCenso, A, Cullum, N & Ciliska, D (1998) Implementing evidence-based nursing: some misconceptions. *Evidence-Based Nursing* 1 (2) 38–39

Disability Rights Commission (2006) *Are we taking the dis?* available at www.drc.org.uk/disability debate

Dooris, M (2001) *Health promoting universities: policy and practice: a UK perspective.* CCPH 2001 conference papers, available at www.depts.washington.edu/ccph/pdf_files/p-dooris.pdf

Dooris, M (2005) Healthy settings: challenges to generating evidence of effectiveness. *Health Promotion International* 21 (1) 55–65

Dooris, M & Thompson, J (2001) Health-promoting universities: an overview, pp. 156–168 in Scriven, A & Orme, J (2001) *Health promotion professional perspectives.* Palgrave, Basingstoke

Downie, R S, Fyfe, C & Tannahill, A (1992) *Health promotion: models and values.* Oxford University Press, Oxford

Duan, N, Fox, S, Pitkin, K, Derose, K, Carson, S & Stockdale, S (2005) Identifying churches for community-based mammography promotion: lessons from the LAMP study. *Health Education and Behaviour* 32 (4) 536–548

Duffy, M (2000) The Internet as a research and dissemination resource. *Health Promotion International* 15 (4) 349–353

Duffy, M, Wimbush, E, Reece, J & Eadie, D (2002) Net profits? Web site development and health improvement. *Health Education* 103 (5) 278–285, available at www.emeraldinsight.com

Dunne, C & Somerset, M (2004) Health promotion in university: what do students want? *Health Education* 104 (6) 360–370

Duval, B, Serre, G, de Shadmani, R, Boulainne, N, Pohani, G, Naus, M, Rochette, L, Fradet, M D, Kain, C F & Ward, B J (2003) A population based comparison between travellers who consulted travel clinics and those who did not. *Journal of Travel Medicine* 10 (1) 4–10

Dyer, K J, Fearon, K L H, Buckner, K & Richardson, R A (2005) Diet and colectoral cancer risk: evaluation of a nutritional leaflet. *Health Education Journal* 64 (3) 247–55

Elder, J P (2001) *Behaviour change and public health in the developing world.* Sage, London

Ellis, A & Beattie, G (1986) The psychology of language and communication. Laurence Erlbaum, London

Eng, T R (2004) Population health technologies: emerging innovations for the health of the American public. *Journal of Preventive Medicine* 26 (3) 237–242

Evans, W D, Wasserman, J, Bertolotti, E & Martine, S (2002) Branding behaviour: the strategy behind the truth campaign. *Social Marketing Quarterly* VIII (3) 17–29

Ewles, L & Simnett, I (2003) *Promoting health: a practical guide,* 5th edition. Bailliere Tindall, London

Eysenbach, G (2001) What is e-health? *Journal of Medical Internet Research* 3 (2), available at www.jmir.org/2001/2/e20/

Ezedinachi, E N U, Ross, M W, Meremiku, M, Essien, E J, Edem, C B, Ekure, E & Ita, O (2002) The impact of an intervention to change health workers HIV/AIDS attitudes and knowledge in Nigeria: a controlled trial. *Public Health* 116 (2)106–112

Farr, A C, Witte, K & Jarato, K (2005) The effectiveness of media use in health education: evaluation of a HIV/AIDS radio campaign in Ethiopia. *Journal of Health Communication* 10 (3) 225–235

Farrelly, M C, Niederdeppe, J & Yarsevich, J (2003) Youth tobacco prevention mass media campaigns: past, present, and future directions. *Tobacco Control* 12 (Suppl 1) i35–i47

Fernando, S (2003) *Cultural diversity, mental health and psychiatry.* Routledge, London

Food Standards Agency (2006) *Salt – eat no more than 6g a day,* available at http://www.salt.gov.uk

Fors, M & Moreno, A (2002) The benefits and obstacles of implementing ICTs strategies for development from a bottom-up approach. *Aslib proceedings* 54 (3) 198–206, available at www.emeraldinsight.com

Fotheringham, M J, Owies, D, Leslie, E & Owen, N (2000) Interactive health communication in preventive medicine: Internet-based strategies in teaching and research. *American Journal of Preventive Medicine* 19 (2) 113–120

Freudenberg, N (2005) Public health advocacy to change corporate practices: implications for health education practice and research. *Health Education and Behaviour* 32 (3) 298–319

Gainer, E, Sollet, C, Ulmann, M, Levy, D & Ulmann, A (2003) Surfing on the morning after: analysis of an emergency contraception website. *Contraception* 67 (3) 195–199

Gerrish, K (2000) Individual care: its conceptualisation and practice within a multiethnic society. *Journal of Advanced Nursing* 32 (1) 91–99

Giles, A (ed.) (2003) *A life-course approach to coronary heart disease prevention: scientific and policy review.* The Stationery Office, London

Giles, M, McClenahan, C, Cairns, E & Mallet, J (2004) The application of the theory of planned behaviour to blood donation: the importance of self-efficacy. *Health Education Research* 19 (4) 580–591

Glang, A, Noell, J, Ary, D & Swartz, L (2005) Using interactive multimedia to teach pedestrian safety: an exploratory study. *American Journal of Health Behaviour* 29 (5) 435–442

Graff, M, Davies, J & McNorton, M (2004) Cognitive style and cross-cultural differences in Internet use and computer attitudes. *European Journal of Open, Distance and E-Learning* (II), available at www.eurodl.org

Graham, W, Smith, P, Kamal, A, Fitzmaurice, A, Smith, N & Hamilton, N (2000) Randomised controlled trial comparing effectiveness of touch-screen system with leaflet for providing women with information on prenatal tests. *British Medical Journal* 320 (15 01) 155–60, available at www.bmj.com

Gray, J A M (2001) *Evidence-based health care,* 2nd edition. Churchill Livingstone, London

Green, E C & Witte, K (2006) Can fear arousal in public health campaigns contribute to the decline of HIV prevalence. *Journal of Health Communication* 11 (3) 245–259

Green, J (1994) *Talking with children: report to the city advisory board Newcastle Upon-Tyne.* Social Welfare Research Unit, University of Northumbria, Newcastle

Grier, S & Bryant, C A (2005) Social marketing in public health. *Annual Review Public Health* 26 (1) 319–39

Grilli, R, Ramsey, C & Minozzi, S (2006) Mass media interventions: effects in health services utilisation (review). *The Cochrane Library* Issue 1, available at www.thecochranelibrary.com

Guilera, M, Fuentes, M, Grifols, M, Ferrer, J & Badia, X (2006) Does an educational leaflet improve self-reported adherence to therapy in osteoporosis? The OPTIMA study. *Osteoporosis International* 17 (5) 664–671

Hale, J L & Dillard, J P (1995) Fear appeals in health promotion campaigns: too much, too little, or just right? pp. 65–80 in Maibach, E & Parrott, R L *Designing health messages.* Sage, London

Hall, J & Visser, A (2000) Health communication in the century of the patient (Editorial). *Patient Education and Counselling* 41, 115–116

Harari, S, Goodyer, L, Anderson, C & Meyer, J (1997) Cardio: interactive multimedia health promotion software for community pharmacy. *Nutrition and Food Science* 97 (2) 71–75

Harrabin, R, Coote, A & Allen, J (2003) *Health in the news.* Kings Fund Publications, London, available at www.kingsfund.org.uk/publications

Harrison, T (2003) Evidence-based multidisciplinary public health, pp. 228–245 in Orme, J, Powell, J, Taylor, P, Harrison, T & Grey, M (eds) *Public health for the 21st century.* OUP, Buckingham

Havering Primary Care Trust (2004) *Local initiatives and services,* available at www.haveringpct.nhs.uk

Havighurst, R J (1963) Successful ageing, pp. 299–320 in Williams, R H, Tibbetts, C & Donahue, W (eds) *Processes of aging.* Atherton, New York

Hawe, P, Degeling, D & Hall, J (1990) *Evaluating Health Promotion.* MacLennon and Petty, Sydney

Health Development Agency (2004) *The effectiveness of public health campaigns.* HDA Briefing 7 June

Health Development Agency (2005) *HDA evidence base, process and quality standards manual for evidence briefings,* 3rd edition. Health Development Agency, London

Health Protection Agency (2003) *HIV and other STIs in the United Kingdom in 2002: annual report.* Health Protection Agency, London

Health Promotion Agency (NI) (2004) *Breastfeeding. Good for baby. Good for mum,* available at www.healthpromotionagency.org.uk

Health Promotion Unit (Ireland) (2006) *Alcohol awareness campaign – less is more,* available at www.healthpromotion.ie/campaigns/

Help Age International (2002) *State of the world's older people 2002.* Help Age International Publication, available at www.helpage.org

Henley, N & Donovan, R J (2003) Young people's responses to death threat appeals: do they really feel immortal? *Health Education Research* 18 (1) 1–14

Hill, L (2004) *Alcohol promotion via mass media: the evidence on (in)effectiveness.* Eurocare 'Bridging the Gap' conference report, Warsaw, available at www.eurocare.org

Hong, T (2006) Contributing factors to the use of health-related websites. *Journal of Health Communication* 11 (2) 149–165

Hopman-Rock, M, Bourghouts, J A J & Leurs, M T W (2004) Determinants of participation in a health education and exercise program on television. *Preventive Medicine* 41 (3), 232–239

Huhman, M, Heitzler, C & Wong, F (2004) The VERB™ campaign logic model: a tool for planning and evaluation. *Preventing Chronic Disease (serial online)* 1 (3), available at www.cdc.gov/pcd/issues/2004/jul/04_0633.htm

Humphris, G M & Field, E A (2004) An oral health information leaflet for two smokers in primary care: results from two randomised control trials. *Community Dentistry and Oral Epidemiology* 32 (2) 143–9

Hussain, A, Aaro, L E, Kvale, G (1997) Impact of a health education program to promote consumption of vitamin A rich foods in Bangladesh. *Health Promotion International* 12 (2) 103–109

Iliffe, S, Kharicha, K, Harari, D, Swift, C & Stuck, A E (2005) Health risk appraisal for older people in general practice using an expert system: a pilot study. *Health and Social Care in the Community* 13 (1) 21–29

Israel, M & Chui, W H (2006) If 'something works' is the answer what is the question: supporting pluralist evaluation in community corrections in the United Kingdom. *European Journal of Criminology* 3, 181–200

Jackson, C, Lawton, R, Knapp, P, Raynor, D K, Connor, M, Lowe, C & Closs, S J (2005) Beyond intention: do specific plans increase health behaviours in patients in primary care? A study of fruit and vegetable consumption. *Social Science and Medicine* 60, 2383–2381

Jackson, I D & Duffy, B K (eds) (1998) *Health communication research.* Westport Court, Greenwood

Jacobs, E A, Karavolos, K, Rathouz, P J, Ferris, T G & Powell, L H (2005) Limited English proficiency and breast and cervical screening in a multi-ethnic population. *American Journal of Public Health* 95 (8) 1410–1416

Jamieson, A (2002) Theory and practice in social gerontology, pp. 7–20 in Jamieson, A & Victor, C *Researching ageing and later life.* Open University Press, Buckingham

Janz, N K & Becker, M H (1984) The health belief model a decade later. *Health Education Quarterly* 11 (1) 1–47

Jary, D & Jary, J (1991) *Dictionary of Sociology.* Harper Collins, London

Johnstone, H (1999) Lessons from the experience in the sexual health service at Thameside Community Health care NHS trust. *Bandolier* 3, available at www.jr2.ac.uk/bandolier

Jones, L, Siddell, M & Douglas, J (eds) (2002) *The challenges of promoting health: exploration and action* 2nd edition. Open University Press, Basingstoke

Jones, S & Donovan, R J (2004) Does theory inform practice in health promotion in Australia? *Health Education Research* 19 (1) 1–14

Joseph Rowntree Foundation (2003) *An evaluation of a young disabled people's peer mentoring/support project,* available at www.jrf.org.uk

Kakai, H, Maskarinec, G, Shumay, D M Tatsumura, Y & Tasaki, K (2003) Ethnic difference in choices of health information by cancer patients using complementary and alternative medicine: an exploratory study with correspondence analysis. *Social Science and Medicine* 56 (2) 851–862

Kane, S & Kirby, M (2002) Wealth, poverty and welfare. Palgrave, Basingstoke

Kaphingst, K, Dejong, W, Rudd, R & Daltroy, L (2004) A content analysis of direct to consumer television prescription drug advertisements. *Journal of health communication* 9 (6) 515–528

Katz, J, Perbedy, A & Douglas, J (eds) (2000) *Promoting health: knowledge and practice*. Open University Press, Basingstoke

Kelley, K & Abraham, C (2004) RCT of a theory-based intervention promoting healthy eating and physical activity amongst out-patients older than 65 years. *Social Science and Medicine* 59 (4) 787–797

Kelman, H (1961) Processes of opinion change. *Public Opinion Quarterly* 25, 57–78

Kidd, P, Reed, D, Weaver, L, Westnear, S & Rayens, M K (2003) The transtheoretical model of change in adolescents: implications for injury prevention. *Journal of Safety Research* 34 (3) 281–288

Kiger, A (2004) *Teaching for health*, 3rd edition. Churchill Livingstone, London

King, R, Estey, J, Allen, S, Kegeles, S, Wolf, W, Valentine, C & Sefulira, A (1995) A family planning intervention to reduce vertical transmission of HIV in Rwanda. *AIDS* 9 (Suppl 1) 45–51

Kirigia, J M, Seddoh, A, Gatwiri, D, Muthuri, L H K & Seddoh, J (2005) E-health: determinants, opportunities, challenges and the way forward for countries in the WHO Africa region. *BMC Public Health* 5 (137), available at www.biomedcentral.com/1471-2458/5/137

Kiyu, A, Steinkuehler, A, Hashim, J, Hall, J, Lee, P & Taylor, R (2006) Evaluation of the healthy village programme in Kapit district Sarawak Malaysia. *Health Promotion International* 21 (1) 13–18

Kobetz, E, Vatalaro, K, Moore, A & Earp, J A (2005) Taking the transtheoretical model into the field: a curriculum for lay health advisors. *Health Promotion Practice* 6 (3) 329–337

Korp, P (2006) Health on the Internet: implications for health promotion. *Health Education Research* 21 (1) 78–86

Kotler, P, Roberto, N & Lee, N (2002) *Social marketing: improving the quality of life*. Sage, California

Kreps, G L (2003) The impact of communication on cancer risk, incidence, morbidity, mortality and quality of life. *Health Communication* 15 (2) 161–169

Kreuter, M, Kinner, C, Haire-Joshu, D & Clark, E (1998) *Cultural tailoring for cancer prevention in black women*. Health Communication Research, laboratory, St. Louis

Kreuter, M W, Lukwago, S N, Bucholtz, D C, Clark, E M & Sanders-Thompson, V (2002) Achieving cultural appropriateness in health promotion programs: targeted and tailored approaches. *Health Education and Behaviour* 30 (2) 133–146

Lajunen, T & Räsänen, M (2004) Can social psychological models be used to promote bicycle helmet use among teenagers? A comparison of the health belief model, theory of planned behaviour and the locus of control. *Journal of Safety Research* 35 (1) 115–123

Lancaster, R & Ward, R (2002) *Management of work-related road safety*, for HSE/Scottish Executive. The Stationery Office, Norwich, available at www.hse.gov.uk

Lavin, D & Groarke, A (2005) Dental-floss behaviour: a test of the predictive utility of the theory of planned behaviour and the effects of making implementation interventions. *Psychology, Health and Medicine* 10 (3) 243–252

Lee, R G & Garvin, T (2003) Moving from information transfer to information exchange in health and health care. *Social Science and Medicine* 56 (3) 449–464

Leiner, M, Handal, G & Williams, D (2004) Patient communication: a multi-disciplinary approach using animated cartoons. *Health Education Research* 19 (5) 591–595

Lenaghan, J (ed) (1998) *Rethinking IT health*. Institute for Public Policy Research. London

Levandowski, B A, Sharma, P, Lane, S D, Webster, N, Nestor, A M, Cibula, D A & Huntington, S (2006) Parental literacy and infant health: an evidence-based health start intervention. *Health Promotion Practice* 7 (1) 95–102

Lewin, K (1951) *Field theory in social science: selected theoretical papers*. Harper Row, New York

Lewis, R K & Green, B L (2000) Assessing the health attitudes, beliefs and behaviours of Africa Americans attending church: a comparison from two communities. *Journal of Community Health* 25 (3) 211–224

Lewis, Y R, Shain, L, Quinn, S C, Turner, K & Moore, T (2002) Building community trust: lessons from an STD/HIV peer educator program with African American barbers and beauticians. *Health Promotion Practice* 3 (2) 133–143

Lieberman, D A (2001) Using interactive media in communication campaigns for children and adolescents, pp. 373–388 in Rice, R E & Aktin, C K (eds) *Public communication campaigns*, 3rd edition. Sage, California

Lin, P, Simoni, J M & Zemon, V (2005) The health belief model, sexual behaviours, and HIV risk among Taiwanese immigrants. *Aids Education and Research* 17 (5) 469–83

Linnan, L A, Kim, A E, Wasilewski, Y, Lee, A M, Yang, J, Solomon, F (2001) Working with licensed cosmetologists to promote health: results from the North Carolina BEAUTY and health pilot study. *Preventive Medicine* 33, 606–612

Linnan, L A, Owens Ferguson, Y, Wasilewski, Y, Lee, A M, Yang, J, Solomon, F & Katz, M (2005) Using community-based participatory research methods to reach women with health messages: results from the North Carolina BEAUTY and health pilot project. *Health Promotion Practice* 6 (2) 164–173

Lowell, S L & Ziglio, E (2003) Health promotion as an investment strategy: a perspective for the 21st century, in Sidell, M, Jones, L, Katz, J, Peberdy, A & Douglas, J (2003) *Debates and dilemmas in promoting health*. Palgrave Macmillan, Basingstoke, p. 412–422

MacDonald, T (1998) *Re-thinking health promotion*. Routledge, London and New York

Macfayden, L, Stead, M & Hastings, G (1999) *A synopsis of social marketing*, available at www.ism.stir.ac.uk/pdf_docs/social_marketing.pdf

Macias, W, Stravchansky Lewis, L & Smith, T L (2005) Health-related message boards/chat rooms on the web: discussion content and implications for pharmaceutical sponsorships. *Journal of Health Communication* 10 (3) 209–223

Marcus, B H, Owen, N, Forsyth, L H, Cavil, N A & Fridinger, F (1998) Physical activity interventions using mass media, print media and IT. *American Journal of Preventive Medicine* 15 (4) 362–378

Markens, S, Fox, S A, Taub, B & Gilbert, M L (2002) Role of black churches in health promotion programs: lessons from the Los Angeles mammography promotion in churches program. *American Journal of Public Health* 92 (5) 805–810

Marks, L (2003) *Evidence-based practice in tackling inequalities in health*. Report of a research and development project, University of Durham, available at www.dur.ac.uk/resources/public.health/publications/

Marr, J & Kershaw, B (1998) *Caring for older people: developing specialist practice*. Arnold, London

Marshall, S J & Biddle, S J H (2001) The transtheoretical model of behaviour change: a meta-analysis of applications to physical activity and exercise. *Annals of Behavioural Medicine* 23 (4) 229–246

Marston, C (2004) Gendered communication among young people in Mexico: implications for sexual health interventions. *Social Science and Medicine* 59 (3) 445–456

Martinson, B E & Hindman, D B (2005) Building a health promotion agenda in local newspapers. *Health Education Research* 20 (1) 51–60

Matteelli, A & Carosi, G (2001) Sexually transmitted diseases in travellers. *Clinical Infectious Disease* 32 (7) 1063–7

Matthews, B (2004) Grey literature: resources for locating unpublished research. *C&RL News* 65 (3)

Maziak, W, Eissenberg, T, Rastam, S, Hammal, F, Asfar, T, Bachir, M, Fouad, M F & Ward, K D (2004) Beliefs and attitudes related to narghile (waterpipe) smoking among university students in Syria. *Journal of Annals of Epidemiology* 14 (9) 646–654

Mbananga, N & Becker, P (2002) Use of technology in reproductive health information designed for communities in South Africa. *Health Education Research* 17 (2) 195–209

McAlister, A L, Gumina, T, Urjanheimo, E L, Laatikainen, T, Uhanov, M, Oganov, R & Puska, P (2000) Promoting smoking cessation in Russian Karelia: a 1-year community based program with quasi-experimental evaluation. *Health Promotion International* 15 (2)109–112

McCoy, M R, Couch, D, Duncan, N D & Lynch, G S (2005) Evaluating an Internet weight-loss program for diabetes prevention. *Health Promotion International* 20 (3) 221–228

McDaniel, A M, Casper, G R, Hutchinson, S K & Stratton, R M (2005) Design and testing of an interactive smoking cessation intervention for inner-city women. *Health Education Research* 20 (3) 379–384

McGuire, W J (1976) Some internal psychological factors influencing consumer choice. *Journal of Consumer Research* 2 (4) 302–319

McGuire, W J (2001) Input and output variables currently promising for constructing persuasive communications, pp. 22–48 in Rice, R E & Aktin, C K (eds) *Public communication campaigns*, 3rd edition. Sage, California

Mckee, I (2003) Rhetorical spaces: participation and pragmatism in the evaluation of health community work. *Evaluation* 3, 307–324

McQueen, D V (2000) Strengthening the evidence base for health promotion. *Health Promotion International* 16 (3) 261–268

McQueen, D V (2002) The evidence debate (Editorial). *Journal of Epidemiology and Community Health* 56, 83–83

Men's Health Forum (2004) *Will there be anything else, sir?* Men's Health Forum Newsletter, March, available at www.menhealthforum.org.uk

Merakou, K & Kourea-Kremastinou, J (2006) Peer education in HIV prevention: an evaluation in schools. *The European Journal of Public Health* 16 (2) 128–132

Metropolitan Police London (2006) *Know what you're getting into,* available at www.met.police.uk

Meyer, G, Roberto, A J, Atkin, C K (2003) A radio-based approach to promoting gun safety: process and outcome evaluation implication and insights. *Health Communication* 15 (3) 299–318

Milburn, K (1995) Critical view of peer education with young people with special reference to sexual health. *Health Education Research* 10 (4) 407–20

Miller, P (2001) *Health economic evaluation: Trent focus for research and development in primary care.* Trent Institute for Health Services Research and Dept of Economics, Nottingham University, Nottingham

Minardi, H & Riley, M (1997) *Communication in health care: a skills-based approach.* Butterworth-Heinemann, London

MIND (2006) *Promoting positive attitudes to mental distress,* available at www.mind.org.uk

Monahan, J L (1995) Thinking positively using positive affect when designing health messages, pp. 81–98 in Maibach, E & Parrott, R L *Designing health messages.* Sage, London

MORI (2005) *Technology tracker.* Technology research information, MORI, available at www.mori.com/technology/techtracker.shtml

Morrell, P. (2001) Social factors affecting communication, pp. 33–44 in Ellis, R B, Gates, R J & Kenworthy, N *Interpersonal communication in nursing.* Churchill Livingstone, London

Moser, R P, Green, V, Weber, D & Doyle, C (2005) Psychosocial correlates of fruit and vegetable consumption among African American men. *Journal of Nutrition Education and Behaviour* 37 (6) 306–14

Mulberry Research and Consulting Group (2004) *Psychological factors affecting transport mode choice* (A64), available at www.imd.dft.gov.uk

Murphy, S & Bennett, P (2002) Psychology and health, ch. 2 in Bunton, R & Macdonald, G (eds) *Health promotion: disciplines, diversity and developments*, 2nd edition. Routledge, London

Myhre, S L & Flora, J A (2000) HIV/AIDS communication campaigns: progress and prospects. *Journal of Health Communication* 5 (Suppl.) 29–45

Naidoo, J & Wills, J (2000) *Health promotion: foundations for practice*, 2nd edition. Baillere Tindall and RCN, London

Naidoo, J & Wills, J (2004) *Public health and health promotion: developing practice.* Bailliere Tindall, London

National No Smoking Day (2006) *National no smoking day,* available at www.nosmokingday.org.uk

National Public Health Service for Wales (2005) *Designed for life: health impacts of tourism in the UK – key findings from literature,* available at www.wales.nhs.uk

National Social Marketing Centre (NSMC) (2006) *Its our health.* NSMC, London, available at www.nsms.org.uk

Neale, J, McKeganey, N, Hay, G & Oliver, J (2001) *Recreational drug use and driving: a qualitative study.* The Scottish Executive Central Research Unit, The Stationery office, Edinburgh, available at www.scotland.gov.uk

Newman, M & Harrier, D (2006) *Teaching and learning resources for evidence-based practice,* available at www.mdx.ac.uk

NHS (2006) *5 a day,* available at www.5aday.nhs.uk

NHS centre for reviews and dissemination (2001) Undertaking systematic reviews of research on effectiveness: CRD'S guidance for those carrying out or commissioning reviews, *CRD report* 4, 2nd edition, available at www.york.ac.uk/inst/crd/report4.htm

NHS Scotland (2003) *DPH annual report 2002,* available at www.thpc.nhs.uk

NICE (2005) *Efficiencies in the guidelines process.* 16 November, available at www.publichealth. nice.org.uk

NICE (2006a) *Public health guidance by topic,* available at www.publichealth. nice.org.uk

NICE (2006b) *Brief interventions and referral for smoking cessation in primary care and other settings,* March, available at www.publichealth.nice.org.uk

Nicholas, D, Huntington, P & Williams, P (2004) The characteristics of users and non-users of a kiosk information system. *Aslib proceedings* 56 (1) 48–61, available at www.emeraldinsight.com

Nishtar, S, Mirza, Y A, Hadi, Y, Badar, A, Yusaf, S & Shahab, S (2004) Newspaper articles as a tool for cardiovascular prevention programs in a developing country. *Journal of Health Communication* 9 (4) 355–369

Noar, S M (2006) A 10-year retrospective of research in health mass media campaigns: where do we go from here? *Journal of Health Communication* 11 (1) 21–42

Norman, P, Conner,. M & Bell, R (2000) The theory of planned behaviour and exercise: evidence for the moderating role of past behaviour. *British Journal of Health Psychology* 5 (3) 249–261

Northouse, L L & Northouse, P G (1998) *Health communication: strategies for health professionals,* 3rd edition. Appleton and Lange, London

Nutbeam, D (1998) Evaluating health promotion: progress problems and solutions. *Health Promotion International* 13 (1) 27–43

Nutbeam, D (1999) The challenge to provide 'evidence' in health promotion (Editorial). *Health Promotion International* 14 (2) 99–101

Nutbeam, D & Smith, C (1993) Maintaining evaluation designs in long term community based health promotion. *Journal of Epidemiology and Community Health* 47, 127–133

O'Hegarty, M, Pederson, L L, Nelson, D F, Mowery, P, Gable, J M & Wortley, P (2006) Reactions of young adult smokers to warning labels on cigarette packages. *American Journal of Preventive Medicine* 30 (6) 467–473

Oemena, A, Brug, J & Lechner, L (2001) Web-based tailored nutrition education: results of a randomised controlled trial. *Health Education Research* 16 (6) 647–660

Office for National Statistics (2001) *Census 2001,* available at www.statistics.gov.uk/census2001/census2001.asp

Office for National Statistics (2004) *Focus on older people overview,* available at www.statistics.gov.uk/focuson/olderpeople

Office for National Statistics (2006) *Internet usage,* available at www.statistics.gov.uk/CCI

Oliver, M (1992) Changing the social relations of research production. *Disability, Handicap and Society* 7 (2) 101–15

O'Malley, A S, Kernes, J F & Johnson, L (1999) Are we getting the message out to all? Health information sources and ethnicity. *American journal of preventative medicine* 17 (3) pp. 198–202

Overseas Development Institute (2006) *Evidence-based policy making,* available at www.odi.org.uk

Papadaki, A, Scott, J A, (2006) Process evaluation of an innovative healthy eating website promoting the Mediterranean diet. *Health Education Research* 21 (2) 206–218

Papauessis, H, Madison, R, Ruygrok, P N, Bassett, S, Harper, T & Gillanders, L (2005) Using the theory of planned behaviour to understand exercise motivation in patients with congenital heart disease. *Psychology, Health and Medicine* 10 (4) 335–343

Parker, E A, Baldwin, G T, Israel, B & Salinas, M (2004) Application of health promotion theories and models for environmental health. *Health Education and Behaviour* 31 (4) 491–509

Pechmann, C & Reibling, E T (2000) *Anti-Smoking advertising* campaigns targeting youth: case studies from USA and Canada. *Tobacco control* 9 (Suppl. ii) ii8–ii31.

Perz, C A, DiClemente, C C & Carbonari, J P (1996) Doing the right thing and the right time? The interaction of stages and processes of change in successful smoking cessation. *Health Psychology* 15 (6) 462–468

Peterson, J, Atwood, J R & Yates, B (2002) Key elements for church-based health promotion programs: outcome-based literature review. *Public Health Nursing* 19 (6) 401–411

Peterson, M, Abraham, A & Waterfield, A (2005) Marketing physical activity: lessons learned from a statewide media campaign. *Health Promotion Practice* 6 (4) 437–446

Platt, S, Gnich, W, Rankin, D, Ritchie, D, Truman J & Backett-Milburn, K (2004) Applying process evaluation: learning from two research projects, pp. 73–89 in Thorogood, M & Coombes, Y (eds) *Evaluating health promotion: practice and methods*, 2nd edition. Oxford University Press, Oxford

Plianbangchang, S (2005) *Keynote address* at the Sixth Global Conference on Health Promotion, Bangkok, 7–11 August, available at www.who.int

Population Communication Services/Centre for Communication Programmes (JHU/CCP) (2003) *A field guide to designing a health communication strategy*, Johns Hopkins University, available at www.eldis.org/Static/Doc18lll.htm

Population Reference Bureau PRB (2005) *Human behaviour holds the key to health improvements worldwide,* available at www.jhuccup.org

Portman Group, The, (2005) *I'll be Des,* available at www.desdriver.co.uk

Pötsönen, R & Kontula, O (1999) How are attitudes towards condom use related to gender and sexual experiences among adolescents in Finland? *Health Promotion International* 14 (3) 211–220

Povlsen, L, Olsen, B & Ladelund, S (2005) Educating families from ethnic minorities in type 1 diabetes – experiences from a Danish intervention study. *Patient Education and Counselling* 59 (2) 164–170

Prochaska, J O & Diclemente, C C (1983) Stages and processes of self-change in smoking: toward an integrative model of change. *Journal of Consulting and Clinical Psychology* 51 (3) 390–395

Provost, S, Gaulin, S, Pipuet-Gauthier, B, Emmanuelli, J, Venne, S, Dion, R, Grenier, J L, Dessau, J & Dubucin (2002) Travel agents and the prevention of health problems among travellers in Quebec. *Journal of Travel Medicine* 9 (1) 3–9

Rada, J, Ratima, M & Howden-Chapman, P (1999) Evidence-based purchasing of health promotion: methodology for reviewing evidence. *Health Promotion International* 14 (2) 177–187

Randolf, W & Viswanath, K (2004) Lessons learned from public health mass media campaigns: marketing health in a crowded media world. *Annual Review of Public Health* 25 (1) 419–37

Raphael, D (2000) The question of evidence in health promotion. *Health Promotion International* 15 (4) 355–367

Reber, A S (1985) *Dictionary of Psychology*. Penguin, London

Reger, B, Cooper, L, Booth-Butterfield, S., Smith, H, Bauman, A, Wootan, M, Middlestadt, S, Marrus, B & Grees, F (2002) Wheeling walks; a community campaign using paid media to encourage walking among sedentary older adults. *Preventive Medicine* 35 (3) 285–292

Reid, L V, Hatch, J & Parrish, T (2003) The role of a historically black university and the black church in community-based health initiatives: the project DIRECT experience. *Journal of Public Health Management Practice* Nov. (Suppl.) S70–73

Reinert, B, Campbell, C, Carver, V & Range, L M (2003) Joys and tribulations of faith-based youth tobacco use prevention: a case study in Mississippi. *Health Promotion Practice* 4 (3) 228–235

Reniscow, K, Jackson, A, Wang, T, De, A K, McCarty, F, Dudley, W & Baranowski, T (2001) A motivational interviewing intervention to increase fruit and vegetable intake through black churches: results of the eat for life trial. *American Journal of Public Health* 91 (10) 1686–1693

Resnicow, K, Jackson, A, Braithwaite, R, Dilorio, C, Blisset, D, Rahotep, S & Periasamy, S (2002) Health body/health spirit: a church-based nutrition and physical activity intervention. *Health Education Research* 17 (5) 562–573

Ribisl, K M (2003) The potential of the Internet as a medium to encourage and discourage youth tobacco use. *Tobacco Control* 12 (Suppl. 1) i48–i59

Ribisl, K, Winkleby, M A, Fortmann, S P & Flora, J A (1998) The interplay of socio-economic status and ethnicity on Hispanic and white men's cardiovascular disease risk and health communication patterns. *Health Education Research* 13 (3) 407–417

Rice, D (2001) The Internet and health communication: a framework of experiences, pp. 5–46 in Rice, R E & Katz, J E (eds) *The Internet and health communication: experiences and expectations*. Sage, London

Rice, R E & Atkin, C K (eds) (2001) *Public communication campaigns,* 3rd edition. Sage, London

Rice, R E & Katz, J E (eds) (2001) *The Internet and health communication. Experiences and expectations.* Sage, London

Risi, L, Bindman, J P, Campbell, O M R, Imrie, J, Everett, K, Bradley, J & Denny, L (2004) Media interventions to increase cervical screening uptake in South Africa: an evaluation of effectiveness. *Health Education Research* 19 (4) 457–468

Robinson, L (2004) Beliefs, values and intercultural communication, pp. 110–120 in Robb, M, Barrett, S, Komaromy, C & Rogers, A (eds) *Communication, relationships and care: a reader.* Routledge, London

Robinson, M (2002) *Communication and health in a multi-ethnic society.* Policy Press, Bristol

Robinson, M & Gilmartin, J (2002) Barriers to communication between health practitioners and service users who are not fluent in English. *Nurse Education Today* 22 (6) 457–465

Rodrigues, R J (2000) Information systems: the key to evidence-based health practice. *Bulletin of the World Health Organization* 78 (11) 1344–1351

Rogers, E (1983) *Diffusion of innovations.* Free Press, New York

Rosengard, C, Adler, N, Gurvey, J E, Dunlop, M B V, Tschann, J M, Millstein, S G & Ellen, J M (2001) Protective role of health values in adolescents' future intentions to use condoms. *Journal of Adolescent Health* 29 (3) 200–207

Rosenstock, I M (1966) Why people use health services. *Milbank Memorial Fund Quarterly* XLIV 3 (2) 94–127

Rosenstock, I M, Stretcher, V J & Becker, M M (1988) Social learning theory and the health belief model, *Health Education Quarterly.* 15 (2) 175–83

Rowe, R & Garcia, J (2003) *Evidence on access to maternity and infant care in England.* National Perinatal Epidemiological Unit, Oxford, available at www.npeau.ox.ac.uk

Russell, C A, Clapp, J D & DeJong, W (2005) Done 4: analysis of a failed social norms marketing campaign. *Health Communication* 17 (1) 57–65

Rutter, D & Quine, L (eds) (2002) *Changing health behaviour.* Open University Press, Buckingham

Ruud, J S, Betts, N, Kritch, K, Nitzke, S, Lohse, B & Boeckner, L (2005) Acceptability of stage-tailored newsletters about fruit and vegetables by young adults. *Journal of the American Dietetic Association* 105 (11) 1774–1778

Rychetnik, L & Wise, M (2004) Advocating evidence-based health promotion: reflections and a way forward. *Health Promotion International* 19 (2) 247–257

Sackett, D, Rosenberg, W, Muir Grey, J A, Hayes, R B & Williamson, W S (1996) Evidence-based medicine: what it is and what it isn't (Editorial). *British Medical Journal* 312, 71–72

Samaritans The, (2006a) *Change our minds 2002 campaign,* available at www.samaritans.org.uk

Samaritans The, (2006b) *txt Samaritans 4 emotional support,* available at www.samaritans.org.uk

Scholten, M (1996) Lost and found: the information-processing model of advertising effectiveness. *Journal of Business Research* 37 (2) 97–104

Scriven, A & Orme, J (2001) Health promotion professionals perspectives. Palgrave, Basingstoke

Seale, C (2002) *Media and health.* Sage, London

Sharp, C (2005) *The improvement of public sector delivery: supporting evidence-based practice through action research,* September, Scottish Executive Research, available at www.scotland.gov.uk/Publications/2005

Shober, J & Farrington, A (1998) *Trent focus for research and development in primary health care: presenting and disseminating research.* Trent Focus, NHS Trent.

Singhal, A & Rogers, E M (2001) The entertainment–education strategy in communication campaigns, pp. 343–356 in Rice, R E & Aktin, C K (eds) *Public communication campaigns*, 3rd edition. Sage, London

Sivaram, S, Johnson, S, Bentley, M E, Go, V F, Lakin, C, Srikishnam, A K, Celentono, K & Solomon, S (2005) Sexual health promotion in Chennai, India: the key role of communication among social networks. *Health Promotion International* 20 (4) 327–333

Smith, B J, Ferguson, C, McKenzie, J, Bauman, A & Vita, D (2002) Impacts from repeated mass media campaigns to promote sun protection in Australia. *Health Promotion International* 17 (1) 51–60

Social Exclusion Unit (1998) *Bringing Britain together: a national strategy for neighbourhood renewal.* The Stationery Office, London

Solomon, F M, Linnan, L A, Wasilewski, Y, Lee, A M, Katz, M I & Yang, J (2004) Observational study in ten beauty salons: results informing development of the North Carolina BEAUTY and health project. *Health Education and Behaviour* 31 (6) 790–807

Solomon, L J & Flynn, B S (2005) Telephone support for pregnant smokers who want to stop smoking. *Health Promotion Practice* 6 (1) 105–108

Sowden, A J & Arblaster, L (2006) Mass media interventions for preventing smoking in young people (Review*). The Cochrane Library* Issue 1, available at www.thecochranelibrary.com

Stead, M, Tagg, S, MacKintosh, A & Eadie, D (2005) Development and evaluation of a mass media theory of planned behaviour intervention to reduce speeding. *Health Education Research* 20 (1) 36–50

Street, R L (2002) Gender difference in health care provider – patient communication: are they due to style, stereotypes, or accommodation? *Patient Education and Counselling* 48 (3) 201–206

Street, R L & Piziak, V K (2001) Improving diabetes care with telecomputing technology, pp. 287–308 in Rice, R E & Katz, J E (eds) *The internet and health communication: experiences and expectations.* Sage, London

Stretcher, V J, Shiffman, S & West, R (2005) Randomised controlled trial of a web-based computer-tailored smoking cessation program as a supplement to nicotine patch therapy. *Addiction* (100) 682–688

Stroke Association (2005) *Stroke is a medical emergency,* available at www.stroke.org.uk

Suggs, L S (2006) A 10-year retrospective of research in new technologies for health communication. *Journal of Health Communication* 11 (1) 61–74

Swann, C J, Falce, C, Morgan, A, Kelly, M, Powell, G, Carmona, C, Taylor, L & Taske, N (2005) *HDA evidence base: process and quality standards manual for evidence briefings,* 3rd edition. Health Development Agency, London

Swinney, J, Anson-Wonkka, C, Maki, E & Corneau, J (2001) Community assessment: a church community and the parish nurse. *Public Health Nursing* 18 (1) 40–44

Tang, K C, Ehsani, J P & McQueen, D V (2003) Evidence-based health promotion: recollections, reflections and reconsiderations. *Journal of Epidemiology and Community Health* 57 (11) 841–843

TeHIP (2005) *The impact of e-health and assistive technologies in health care,* The E-health Innovation Professionals Group, available at www.tehip.org.uk

Thompson, N (2002) *People skills,* 2nd edition. Palgrave Macmillan, Basingstoke

Thorne, S E, Con, A, McGuinness, L, McPherson, G, Harris, S R (2004a) Health care communication issues in multiple sclerosis: an interpretive description. *Qualitative Health Research* 14 (1) 5–22

Thorne, S E, Harris, S R, Mahoney, K, Con A & McGuinness, L (2004b) The context of health care communication in chronic illness. *Patient Education and Counselling* 54 (3) 299–306

Thorne, S E, Nyhlin, K T & Paterson, B L (2000) Attitudes toward patient expertise in chronic illness. *International Journal of Nursing Studies* 37 (4) 303–311

Thorogood, M & Coombes, Y (eds) (2004) *Evaluating health promotion: practice and methods,* 2nd edition. Oxford University Press, Oxford

Thurston, W E & Blundell-Gosselin, H J (2005) The farm as a setting for health promotion: results of a needs assessment in South Central Alberta. *Health and Place* 11, 31–43

Tinker, A (1997) *Older people in modern society.* Longman, London

Tomassini, C (2005) The demographic characteristics of the oldest old in the United Kingdom. *Population Trends* 120, 15–22

Tones, K & Green J (2004) *Health promotion: planning and strategy.* Sage, London

Tones, K & Tilford, S (1994) *Health education: effectiveness, efficiency and equity,* 2nd edition. Chapman & Hall, London

Trifiletti, L B., Gielen, A C, Sleet, D A & Hopkins, K (2005) Behavioural and social sciences theories and models: are they used in unintentional injury prevention research? *Health Education Research* 20 (3) 298–307

Tsouros, A D, Dowding, G, Thompson, J & Dooris, M (eds) (1998) *Health promoting universities, concept experience and framework for action*. WHO, Copenhagen, available at www.who.dk/document/E60163.pdf

UNICEF (2000) Learning from experience: water and environmental sanitation in India. Unicef, available at www.unicef.org/publications/files/pub_wes_en.pdf

US office of discase prevention and health promotion (2000) *Healthy People 2010*, available at www.healthypeople.gov/document/

University of Central Lancashire (2006) *Health settings development unit*, available at www.uclan.ac.uk/facs/health/hsdu/index.htm

Usdin, S, Scheepers, E, Goldstein, S & Japhet, G (2005) Achieving social change on gender-based violence: a report in the impact evaluation of soil cities fourth series. *Social Science and Medicine* 61 (11) 2434–2445

Van Herck, K, Zuckerman, J, Castelli, F, Van Damme, P, Walker, E & Robert, S (2003) Travellers' knowledge, attitudes, and practices on prevention of infectious diseases: results from a pilot study. *Journal of Travel Medicine* 10 (2) 75

Vaughan, P W & Rogers, E M (2000) A stages model of communication effects: evidence from an entertainment–education radio soap opera in Tanzania. *Journal of Health Communication* 5 (3) 203–227

Vydelingum, V (2000) South Asian patients' lived experience of acute care in an English hospital. *Journal of Advanced Nursing* 32 (1)100–107

Walker, A & Maltby, T (1997) *Ageing Europe*. Open University Press, Buckingham

Wallace, S (1998) Telemedicine in the NHS for the millennium and beyond, pp. 55–99 in Lenaghan, J (ed) *Rethinking IT and health*. Institute for Public Policy Research. London

Wallcraft, J (2003) *The mental health service user movement in England*. Sainsbury Centre for Mental Health, London

Wang, S, Moss, J R & Hiller, J E (2005) Applicability and transferability of interventions in evidence-based public health. *Health Promotion International* 21 (1) 76–83

Wardle, J & Huon, G (2000) An experimental investigation of the influences of health information on children's taste preferences. *Health Education Research* 15 (1) 39–44

Watson, K C, Kieckhefer, G M & Olshansky, E (2006) Striving for therapeutic relationships: parent-provider communication in the developmental treatment setting. *Qualitative Health Research* 16 (5) 647–663

Watzlawick, P, Beavin, J & Jackson, D (1967) *The pragmatics of human communication*. Norton, New York

Weinberg, D S, Turner, B J, Wang, H, Myers, R E, & Miller, S (2004) A survey of women regarding factors affecting colorectal cancer screening compliance. *Preventive Medicine* 38 (6) 669–675

Weitkunat, R, Pottgiesser, C, Meyer, N, Crispin, A, Fischer, R, Scotten, K, Keir, J & Überla, K (2003) Perceived risk of bovine spongiform encephalopathy and dietary behaviour. *Journal of Health Psychology* 8 (3) 373–381

West, R (2005) Time for a change: putting the transtheoretical model to rest. (Editorial) *Addiction* 11 (8) 1036–1039

Whitehead, D (2004) The health promoting university (HPU): the role and function of nursing. *Nurse Education Today* 24 (6) 466–472

Whitelaw, S, Baxendale, A, Bryce, C, Machardy, L, Young, I & Witney, E (2001) 'Settings'-based health promotion: a review. *Health Promotion International* 16 (4) 339–353

Wiggers, J, Sanson-Fisher, R (2001) Evidence-based health promotion, pp. 126–145 in Scott, D & Weston, R *Evaluating health promotion*. Nelson Thornes, Cheltenham

Wilder-Smith, A, Khairullah, N S, Song, J H, Chen, C Y & Torresi, J (2003) Travel health knowledge, attitudes and practices among Australasian travellers. *Journal of Travel Medicine* 10 (3) 177

Wong, C & Tang, C S (2005) Practice of habitual and volitional health behaviours to prevent severe acute respiratory syndrome among Chinese adolescents in Hong Kong. *Journal of Adolescent Health* 36 (3) 193–200

World Health Assembly (1998) *Resolution WHA 51.12 on health promotion: agenda item 20*, 16 May, WHO, available at www.who.int

World Health Organisation (1986) *Ottawa charter for health promotion,* 17–21 November, Ottawa, available at www.who.int/hpr/NPH/docs/ottawa_charter_hp. pdf

World Health Organisation (1998) *Health promotion: milestones on the road to a global alliance*, Fact sheet N°171 Revised June 1998, available at www.who.int

World Health Organization (2000) *International classification of impairments, disabilities and handicaps*, WHO, Geneva

World Health Organisation (2003) *Healthy cities around the world: an overview of the healthy cities movement in six WHO regions*, WHO, Belfast, available at www.euro.who.int/document/hcp/healthy cityworld.pdf

World Health Organization (2004) *Global strategy on diet, physical activity and health,* available from www.who.int/dietphysicalactivity/en

Wray, R J, Hornik, R M, Gandy, O H, Stryker, J, Ghez, M & Mitchell-Clark, K (2004) Preventing domestic violence in an African American community: assessing the impact of a dramatic radio serial. *Journal of Health Communication* 9 (11) 31–52

Wright, L (1999) Evaluation in health promotion: the proof of the pudding, in Perkins, E R, Simnett, I & Wright, L (eds) *Evidence-based health promotion*. Wiley, Chichester

Wyatt, J (1998) Four barriers to realising the information revolution in health care, pp. 100–122 in Lenaghan, J (ed) *Rethinking IT and health*. Institute for Public Policy Research, London

Xiangyang, T, Lan, Z, Xueping, M, Tao, Z, Yuzhen, S & Jagusztyn, M (2003) Beijing health promoting universities: practice and evaluation. *Health Promotion International* 18 (2) 107–113

Zondervan, M, Kuper, H, Solomon, A & Buchan, J (2004) Health Promotion for trachoma control. *Community Eye Health Journal* 17 (52) 57–58

Index